Eye Movement Desensitization and Reprocessing (EMDR) Therapy

Theories of Psychotherapy Series

Acceptance and Commitment Therapy
  Steven C. Hayes and Jason Lillis

Adlerian Psychotherapy
  Jon Carlson and Matt Englar-Carlson

*The Basics of Psychotherapy: An Introduction to Theory and Practice,
  Second Edition*
  Bruce E. Wampold

Behavior Therapy
  Martin M. Antony and Lizabeth Roemer

Brief Dynamic Therapy, Second Edition
  Hanna Levenson

Career Counseling, Second Edition
  Mark L. Savickas

Cognitive–Behavioral Therapy, Second Edition
  Michelle G. Craske

Cognitive Therapy
  Keith S. Dobson

Dialectical Behavior Therapy
  Alexander L. Chapman and Katherine L. Dixon-Gordon

Emotion-Focused Therapy, Revised Edition
  Leslie S. Greenberg

Existential–Humanistic Therapy, Second Edition
  Kirk J. Schneider and Orah T. Krug

Eye Movement Desensitization and Reprocessing (EMDR) Therapy
  Mark C. Russell and Francine Shapiro

Family Therapy
  William J. Doherty and Susan H. McDaniel

Feminist Therapy, Second Edition
  Laura S. Brown

Gestalt Therapy
Gordon Wheeler and Lena Axelsson

Interpersonal Psychotherapy
Ellen Frank and Jessica C. Levenson

Narrative Therapy, Second Edition
Stephen Madigan

Person-Centered Psychotherapies
David J. Cain

Psychoanalysis and Psychoanalytic Therapies, Second Edition
Jeremy D. Safran and Jennifer Hunter

Psychotherapy Case Formulation
Tracy D. Eells

Psychotherapy Integration
George Stricker

Rational Emotive Behavior Therapy, Second Edition
Albert Ellis and Debbie Joffe Ellis

Reality Therapy
Robert E. Wubbolding

Relational–Cultural Therapy, Second Edition
Judith V. Jordan

Theories of Psychotherapy Series

Matt Englar-Carlson, Series Editor

Eye Movement Desensitization and Reprocessing (EMDR) Therapy

Mark C. Russell and
Francine Shapiro

AMERICAN PSYCHOLOGICAL ASSOCIATION

Published by
American Psychological Association
750 First Street, NE
Washington, DC 20002
https://www.apa.org

Order Department
https://www.apa.org/pubs/books
order@apa.org

In the U.K., Europe, Africa, and the Middle East, copies may be ordered from Eurospan
https://www.eurospanbookstore.com/apa
info@eurospangroup.com

Typeset in Minion by Circle Graphics, Inc., Reisterstown, MD

Printer: Sheridan Books, Chelsea, MI
Cover Designer: Beth Schlenoff Design, Bethesda, MD
Cover Art: *Lily Rising,* 2005, oil and mixed media on panel in craquelure frame, by Betsy Bauer

Library of Congress Cataloging-in-Publication Data

Names: Russell, Mark C. (Mark Charles), 1960- author. | Shapiro, Francine, author.
Title: Eye movement desensitization and reprocessing (EMDR) therapy /
    by Mark C. Russell and Francine Shapiro.
Description: Washington, DC : American Psychological Association, [2022] |
    Series: Theories of psychotherapy | Includes bibliographical references
    and index.
Identifiers: LCCN 2021026240 (print) | LCCN 2021026241 (ebook) |
    ISBN 9781433836596 (paperback) | ISBN 9781433838460 (ebook)
Subjects: LCSH: Eye movement desensitization and reprocessing. |
    Psychotherapy. | BISAC: PSYCHOLOGY / Psychopathology / Post-Traumatic
    Stress Disorder (PTSD) | PSYCHOLOGY / Physiological Psychology
Classification: LCC RC489.E98 R87 2022 (print) | LCC RC489.E98 (ebook) |
    DDC 616.89/14—dc23
LC record available at https://lccn.loc.gov/2021026240
LC ebook record available at https://lccn.loc.gov/2021026241

https://doi.org/10.1037/0000273-000

Printed in the United States of America

10 9 8 7 6 5 4 3 2 1

Contents

Series Preface   *ix*

How to Use This Book With APA Psychotherapy Videos   *xv*

Acknowledgments   *xvii*

1. Introduction   3

2. History   11

3. Theory   25

4. The Therapy Process   41

5. Evaluation   101

6. Suggestions for Future Developments   127

7. Summary   135

Appendix A: EMDR Therapy Standard Protocol Worksheet   139

Appendix B: Safe and Calm Place Exercise Protocol   145

Appendix C: Resource Development and Installation Protocol   149

Appendix D: Sample of Possible Negative and Positive Cognitions   153

Appendix E: EMDR Therapy Case Example   155

CONTENTS

Glossary of Key Terms   169

Suggested Readings and Resources   171

References   175

Index   195

About the Authors   205

About the Series Editor   207

Series Preface

Matt Englar-Carlson

Some might argue that in the contemporary clinical practice of psychotherapy, the focus on evidence-based intervention and effective outcome has overshadowed theory in importance. Maybe. But at the same time, it is clear that psychotherapists adopt and practice according to one theory or another because their experience, and decades of empirical evidence, suggests that having a sound theory of psychotherapy leads to greater therapeutic success. Theory is fundamental in guiding psychotherapists in understanding *why* people behave, think, and feel in certain ways, and it provides the guidance to then contemplate *what* a client can do to instigate meaningful change. Still, the role of theory in the helping process itself can be hard to explain. This narrative about solving problems may help convey theory's importance:

> Aesop tells the fable of the sun and wind having a contest to decide who was the most powerful. From above the earth, they spotted a person walking down the street, and the wind said that he bet he could get his coat off. The sun agreed to the contest. The wind blew, and the person held on tightly to his coat. The more the wind blew, the tighter the person held on to his coat. The sun said it was his turn. He put all of his energy into creating warm sunshine, and soon the person took off his coat.

What does a competition between the sun and the wind to get the person to remove a coat have to do with theories of psychotherapy? This deceptively simple story highlights the importance of theory as the precursor to any effective intervention—and hence to a favorable outcome. Without a guiding theory, a psychotherapist might treat the symptom without understanding the role of the individual. Or we might create power conflicts with our clients and not understand that, at times, indirect means of helping (sunshine) are often as effective as—if not more so than—direct ones (wind). In the absence of theory, a psychotherapist might lose track of the treatment rationale and instead get caught up in, for example, social correctness and not wanting to do something that looks too simple.

What exactly *is* theory? The *APA Dictionary of Psychology, Second Edition* defines theory as "a principle or body of interrelated principles that purports to explain or predict a number of interrelated phenomena" (VandenBos, 2015, p. 1081). In psychotherapy, a theory is a set of principles used to explain human thought and behavior, including what causes people to change. In practice, a theory frames the goals of therapy and specifies how to pursue them. Haley (1997) noted that a theory of psychotherapy ought to be simple enough for the average psychotherapist to understand but comprehensive enough to account for a wide range of eventualities. Furthermore, a theory guides action toward successful outcomes while generating hope in both the psychotherapist and client that recovery is possible.

Theory is the compass that allows psychotherapists to navigate the vast territory of clinical practice. In the same ways that navigational tools have been modified to adapt to advances in thinking and ever-expanding territories to explore, theories of psychotherapy have evolved over time to account for advances in science and technology. The different schools of theories are commonly referred to as *waves*—the first wave of psychodynamic theories (i.e., Adlerian, psychoanalytic), the second wave of learning theories (i.e., behavioral, cognitive-behavioral), the third wave of humanistic theories (i.e., person centered, gestalt, existential), the fourth wave of feminist and multicultural theories, and the fifth wave of postmodern and constructivist theories (i.e., narrative, constructivist). In many ways, these waves represent how psychotherapy has adapted and responded to changes in psychology, society, and epistemology, as well as to changes in the nature of psychotherapy itself. The wide variety of theories is also a testament to the different ways in which the same human behavior can be conceptualized depending on the view one espouses (Frew & Spiegler, 2012). Our theories of psychotherapy are also challenged to expand beyond the primarily Western worldview endemic in most psychotherapy theories and the practice of psychotherapy itself. That revision and correction requires theories and psychotherapists to become more inclusive of the full range of human diversity to reflect an understanding of human behavior that accounts for a client's context, identity, and intersectionality (American Psychological Association, 2017). To that end, psychotherapy and the theories that guide it are dynamic and responsive to the changing world around us.

With these two concepts in mind—the central importance of theory and the natural evolution of theoretical thinking—the APA Theories of Psychotherapy Series was developed. This series was created by my father (Jon Carlson) and me. Although educated in different eras, we both had a love of theory and often spent time discussing the range of complex ideas that drove each model. Even though my father identified strongly as an Adlerian and I was parented and raised from the Adlerian perspective, my father always espoused an appreciation for other theories and theorists— and that is something I picked up from him. As university faculty members teaching courses on the theories of psychotherapy, we wanted to create learning materials that not only highlighted the essence of the major theories for professionals and professionals in training but also clearly brought the reader up-to-date on the current status of the models, future directions with an emphasis on the inclusive application of the theories with clients representing the range of identities. Often in books on theory, the biography of the original theorist overshadows the evolution of the model. In contrast, our intent was to highlight the contemporary uses of the theories as well as their history and context—both past and present.

As this project began, we faced two immediate decisions: which theories to address and who best to present them. We assessed graduate-level theories of psychotherapy courses to see which theories are being taught, and we explored popular scholarly books, articles, and conferences to determine which theories draw the most interest. We then developed a dream list of authors from among the best minds in contemporary theoretical practice. To that end, each author in the series is one of the leading proponents of that approach as well as a knowledgeable practitioner. We asked each author to review the core constructs of the theory, bring the theory into the modern sphere of clinical practice by looking at it through a context of evidence-based practice, and clearly illustrate how the theory looks in application.

This is the 24th title in the series, and many titles are now in their second edition. Each title can stand alone or can be put together with a few other titles to create materials for a course in psychotherapy theories. This option allows instructors to create a course featuring the approaches they believe are the most salient today. To support this end, APA Books has also developed a video for each of the approaches to demonstrate the theory in practice with a real client. Many of the videos show psychotherapy over six sessions with the same client. Contact APA Books for a complete list of available video programs (https://www.apa.org/pubs/videos).

A theories of psychotherapy book series has to address the range of theories—from those reflecting the origin of psychotherapy itself to emerging approaches that seemingly do not fit into any preexisting school of thought. Eye movement desensitization and reprocessing (EMDR) therapy certainly fits into the latter category. The interest in EMDR is clearly associated with the broader understanding in the past 40 years about trauma and trauma treatment. EMDR uniquely presented an alternative way to treat trauma that did not rely on the use of psychopharmacology or traditional approaches to talk therapy. Understandably so, EMDR quickly attracted its share of critics and disciples. In this monograph, Mark C. Russell and Francine Shapiro chronicle the origins and advancement of EMDR. The reader will learn about the core concept, course of treatment, and the expanding evidence base that makes EMDR one of the most sought-after treatments for trauma-associated distress. Sadly, this monograph also represents one of Francine Shapiro's final publications. As the originator of EMDR, Francine's involvement in this monograph was paramount. I had the pleasure of meeting Francine many times, and my father enjoyed his interactions and projects with her, often sharing with me the extent to which her work dazzled him. When the decision was made to include EMDR in this monograph series, I was so pleased with Francine's involvement. I am thankful that Mark continued with this monograph. My appreciation extends to the care and clarity with which Mark presented EMDR in both theory and application, but I am grateful also because now my own graduate students will stop asking me when will this theory series include EMDR.

REFERENCES

American Psychological Association. (2017). *Multicultural guidelines: An ecological approach to context, identity, and intersectionality.* http://www.apa.org/about/policy/multicultural-guidelines.pdf

Frew, J., & Spiegler, M. (2012). *Contemporary psychotherapies for a diverse world* (1st rev. ed.). Routledge.

Haley, J. (1997). *Leaving home: The therapy of disturbed young people.* Routledge.

VandenBos, G. (2015). *APA dictionary of psychology* (2nd ed.). American Psychological Association.

How to Use This Book With APA Psychotherapy Videos

Each book in the Theories of Psychotherapy Series is specifically paired with a video that demonstrates the theory applied in actual therapy with a real client. Many videos feature the author of the book as the guest therapist, allowing students to see an eminent scholar and practitioner putting the theory they write about into action.

The video programs have a number of features that make them excellent tools for learning more about theoretical concepts:

- Many video programs contain six full sessions of psychotherapy over time, giving viewers a chance to see how clients respond to the application of the theory over the course of several sessions.
- Each program has a brief introductory discussion recapping the basic features of the theory behind the approach demonstrated. This allows viewers to review the key aspects of the approach about which they have just read.
- The videos feature volunteer clients in unedited psychotherapy sessions. This provides a unique opportunity to get a sense of the look and feel of real psychotherapy, something that written case examples and transcripts sometimes cannot convey.

The books and videos together make a powerful teaching tool for showing how theoretical principles affect practice. In the case of this book, the video *EMDR for Trauma: Eye Movement Desensitization and Reprocessing,* which features the second author as the guest expert, provides a vivid example of how this approach looks in practice.

For more information, please visit APA Videos at https://www.apa.org/pubs/videos/.

Acknowledgments

As a graduate student in 1990–1991, I (M. C. R.) had the great fortune to serve as Francine Shapiro's research assistant. My meager contributions to this monograph are dedicated to my mentor, my inspiration, my colleague, and my friend, Francine Shapiro, who tragically passed away on June 16, 2019, after a long, courageous battle with cancer. True to form, Francine worked on this book right up to the time of her death.

We express our deepest gratitude to the American Psychological Association and the editors of the Theories of Psychotherapy Series, Matt Englar-Carlson and his late father, Jon Carlson, for their steadfast support of eye movement desensitization and reprocessing (EMDR) as an accepted therapeutic modality worthy of their highly respected series. On a personal note, I (M. C. R.) also wish to acknowledge the unwavering critical support received by the likes of Howard Lipke, Steven Silver, Robbie Dunton, Andrew Leeds, and Charles Figley, as well as my wonderful partner and wife, Mika Russell.

Unfortunately, Dr. Shapiro died before authoring acknowledgments for this book. Dr. Shapiro's latest previous writing was the third edition of her EMDR text *Eye Movement Desensitization and Reprocessing (EMDR) Therapy*, published by Guilford Press in 2018. In her book, Dr. Shapiro offers many poignant acknowledgments worth repeating, including the following:

> Introducing an innovation to the psychology community is notoriously difficult, but we have been blessed with an expanding circle of

openhearted, masterful therapists and researchers, whose ability and integrity reassure me that we are on the right path. To those EMDR therapy trainers, facilitators, and therapists who had the vision to try something new and the courage to spread the word about their experiences—although it may seem like hubris to thank you for things you did out of a sense of personal responsibility and purpose—I am endlessly grateful. Finally, for providing his scientific rigor, patience, and unswerving support, I (F. S.) thank my husband, Bob Welch. (p. xvi)

Eye Movement Desensitization and Reprocessing (EMDR) Therapy

1

Introduction

Eye movement desensitization and reprocessing (EMDR) therapy erupted onto the psychotherapy landscape 32 years ago (F. Shapiro, 1989). EMDR therapy is considered an integrative client-centered psychotherapy emphasizing the brain's information processing system and memories of disturbing events as the bases of psychopathology (F. Shapiro, 2018). By "integrative," we mean that EMDR therapists will routinely observe phenomena such as free association, insight, abreaction, present conflicts linked to unresolved memories, somatic representations of psychological conflict, desensitization effects, the importance of cognitions, and meaning making all within the context of a highly person-centered and neuropsychological approach. Specifically, EMDR therapy emphasizes working with imagery, cognitions, emotions, somatic sensations, and behavior linked to the disturbing memory, as well as attending to past, current, and future-oriented experiential contributors. It is a treatment that focuses on experiences contributing both to pathology and resilience.

https://doi.org/10.1037/0000273-001
Eye Movement Desensitization and Reprocessing (EMDR) Therapy, by M. C. Russell and F. Shapiro

I (F. S.) introduced the treatment in 1987 as eye movement desensitization (EMD), primarily a counterconditioning technique informed by behavioral theory that used clients' eye movements while tracking the therapist's rapid, left-to-right hand gestures to elicit desensitization. My (1989) inaugural study with 22 trauma survivors, including several Vietnam War veterans, revealed the potential for a significant reduction of posttraumatic stress disorder (PTSD) symptoms after a single EMD session, maintained at 3-month follow-up. However, in 1990, I added "reprocessing" to EMD to better account for the broad and often rapid information processing changes believed to exceed mainstream cognitive behavior therapy theoretical explanations (F. Shapiro, 2018). By rejecting an established paradigm for an untested, "accelerated" information processing (AIP) theory, coupled with restrictive training requirements, a 30-year-long controversy has ensued with profound implications. The history and underlying theory of EMDR are described in Chapters 2 and 3 of this book, respectively.

EIGHT PHASES OF THE STANDARD EMDR TRAUMA-FOCUSED PROTOCOL

The standard EMDR protocol reflects an integrative psychotherapy consisting of eight stages as outlined in Table 1.1 and described in some detail in Chapter 4. A key aspect of the eight phases of EMDR can be likened to a series of "checks and balances," whereby the extent of adaptive reprocessing is sequentially reassessed by the inclusion of disparate elements and time dimensions of human experience.

EMDR THERAPY IS AN EVIDENCE-BASED TREATMENT

Since its inception, a total of 36 randomized controlled trials have established the efficacy of EMDR therapy. A summary of EMDR therapy research on traumatized adults and children and other selected clinical populations is provided in Chapter 5. Consequently, EMDR therapy is broadly recognized as an evidence-based treatment for PTSD by every

Table 1.1

Overview of Eight Phases of EMDR Therapy

Phase	Purpose	Procedures
Phase 1: Client history	Obtain background information. Determine suitability for EMDR therapy. Identify reprocessing targets from positive and negative events in client's life.	Administer standard history-taking questionnaires and diagnostic psychometrics. Review criteria and resources. Ask questions regarding (a) past events that have laid the foundation for the pathology, (b) current triggers, and (c) future needs.
Phase 2: Preparation	Prepare appropriate clients for EMDR processing of target memories. Stabilize and increase access to positive affects (calm and safe place).	Educate regarding the symptom picture. Teach metaphors and techniques that foster stabilization and a sense of personal self-mastery and control.
Phase 3: Assessment	Access the target for EMDR processing by stimulating primary components of the memory.	Elicit the image, negative cognition currently held, desired positive belief, current emotions, and physical sensations and obtain baseline measures.
Phase 4: Desensitization	Process experiences toward an adaptive resolution (0 SUD level). Fully process all channels of association to allow a complete assimilation of memories. Incorporate templates for positive experiences.	Use standardized EMDR protocols, allowing the spontaneous emergence of insights, emotions, physical sensations, and other memories. Use "cognitive interweave" to open blocked processing by elicitation of more adaptive information.
Phase 5: Installation	Increase connections to positive adaptive networks. Increase generalization effects within associated memories.	Identify the best positive cognition (initial or emergent). Enhance the validity of the desired positive belief to a 7 validity of cognition.
Phase 6: Body scan	Complete processing of any residual somatic disturbance associated with the target memory.	Concentrate on and process any residual physical sensations.

(continues)

	Table 1.1	
Overview of Eight Phases of EMDR Therapy (*Continued*)		
Phase	Purpose	Procedures
Phase 7: Closure	Ensure client stability at the completion of an EMDR session and between sessions.	Use guided imagery or self-control techniques, if needed. Brief client regarding expectations and behavioral reports between sessions.
Phase 8: Reevaluation	Evaluate treatment effects. Ensure comprehensive processing over time.	Explore what has emerged since last session. Access memory from last session. Evaluate integration within larger social system.

Note. SUD = subjective units of disturbance. From *The EMDR Approach to Psychotherapy: EMDR Humanitarian Assistance Program Basic Training Course* (Part II, p. 6), by F. Shapiro, 2011, EMDR Humanitarian Assistance Program. Copyright 2011 by Francine Shapiro. Reprinted with permission.

major domestic and international practice guideline for traumatic stress injuries, including the following.

United States PTSD Clinical Practice Guidelines

American Psychiatric Association. (2009). *Practice guideline for the treatment of patients with acute stress disorder and posttraumatic stress disorder.* https://psychiatryonline.org/pb/assets/raw/sitewide/practice_guidelines/guidelines/acutestressdisorderptsd.pdf

American Psychological Association. (2017). *Clinical practice guideline for the treatment of PTSD in adults.* https://www.apa.org/ptsd-guideline

Department of Veterans Affairs and Department of Defense. (2017). *VA/DoD clinical practice guideline for the management of post-traumatic stress disorder and acute stress disorder* (Office of Quality and Performance publication 10Q-CPG/PTSD-04/10). Veterans Health Administration, Department of Veterans Affairs and Health Affairs, Department of Defense.

Substance Abuse and Mental Health Services Administration. (2010, October). *Eye movement desensitization and reprocessing.* National Registry of Evidence-Based Programs and Practices, U.S. Department of Health and Human Services.

International PTSD Clinical Practice Guidelines

Bisson, J. I., Roberts, N. P., Andrew, M., Cooper, R., & Lewis, C. (2013). Psychological therapies for chronic post-traumatic stress disorder (PTSD) in adults. *Cochrane Database of Systematic Reviews, 12*(12), Article CD003388. https://doi.org/10.1002/14651858.CD003388.pub4

CREST. (2003). *The management of post-traumatic stress disorder in adults.* Clinical Resource Efficiency Support Team, Northern Ireland Department of Health, Social Services, and Public Safety.

Dutch National Steering Committee Guidelines Mental Health Care. (2003). *Multidisciplinary guideline: Anxiety disorders.* Quality Institute Health Care CBO/Trimbos Institute.

Forbes, D., Bisson, J. I., Monson, C. M., & Berliner, L. (2020). *Effective treatments for PTSD: Practice guidelines from the International Society for Traumatic Stress Studies* (3rd ed.). Guilford Press.

INSERM. (2004). *Psychotherapy: An evaluation of three approaches.* French National Institute of Health and Medical Research.

Katzman, M. A., Bleau, P., Blier, P., Chokka, P., Kjernisted, K., Van Ameringen, M., Antony, M. M., Bouchard, S., Brunet, A., Flament, M., Grigoriadis, S., Mendlowitz, S., O'Connor, K., Rabheru, K., Richter, P. M., Robichaud, M., Walker, J. R., & the Canadian Anxiety Guidelines Initiative Group. (2014). Canadian clinical practice guidelines for the management of anxiety, posttraumatic stress and obsessive-compulsive disorders. *BMC Psychiatry, 14*(Suppl. 1), S1. https://doi.org/10.1186/1471-244X-14-S1-S1

National Council for Mental Health, Bleich, A., Kotler, M., Kutz, L., & Shaley, A. (2002). *National Council for Mental Health: Guideline for the assessment and professional intervention with terror victims in the hospital and in the community.* Israeli National Council for Mental Health.

National Institute for Health and Care Excellence. (2018). *Post-traumatic stress disorder* (NICE Guideline NG116). https://www.nice.org.uk/guidance/ng116

Park, J. E., Ahn, H. N., & Jung, Y. E. (2016). Prevention and treatment of trauma- and stressor-related disorders: Focusing on psychosocial interventions for adult patients. *Journal of Korean Neuropsychiatric Association, 55*(2), 89–96. https://doi.org/10.4306/jknpa.2016.55.2.89

Phoenix Australia Centre for Posttraumatic Mental Health. (2013). *Australian guidelines for the treatment of acute stress disorder and posttraumatic stress disorder.* https://phoenixaustralia.org/wp-content/uploads/2015/03/Phoenix-ASD-PTSD-Guidelines.pdf

Swedish Agency for Health Technology Assessment and Assessment of Social Services. (2005, November). *Treatment of anxiety disorders: A systematic review* (SBU Yellow Report No. 171/1+2).

World Health Organization. (2013). *Guidelines for the management of conditions specifically related to stress.* https://apps.who.int/iris/bitstream/handle/10665/85119/9789241505406_eng.pdf;jsessionid=F5EB3E2FB9A36EA3B0B150BCA86C454F?sequence=1

According to the World Health Organization (WHO; 2013), EMDR was recommended as a first line of treatment for posttraumatic stress disorder in adults before prescribing selective serotonin reuptake inhibitors and tricyclic antidepressants. Specifically, WHO cited several key advantages of EMDR therapy in that it "does not involve (a) detailed descriptions of the traumatic event(s), (b) direct challenging of beliefs, (c) extended exposure, or (d) homework" (p. 1), resulting in its identification as a top-tier trauma-focused psychotherapy.

THE NEED FOR TRAINING

We both firmly believe that clients are best served by therapists informed by research and open to learning new information, expanding their skills, and thinking outside the box. From its inception, therapists and researchers have been strongly encouraged to seek out appropriate training in EMDR therapy. Such training is available worldwide. The EMDR Institute and EMDR International Association (EMDRIA; a 501(c)(6) nonprofit professional organization) were established to develop and monitor EMDR therapy training and practice standards. Regional and national EMDR associations across North and South America, Europe, the Middle East, and Asia have been formed and repeat the call to adhere to the EMDRIA-approved training guidelines. Research has demonstrated the importance of treatment fidelity to the EMDR therapy protocol to obtain the best clinical results possible (Maxfield & Hyer, 2002). An EMDR treatment fidelity rating scale has also been developed to help assess therapeutic integrity to the standard EMDR therapy protocol (Korn et al., 2017).

The American Psychological Association's *Ethical Principles of Psychologists and Code of Conduct* (2017b) stipulates that training and supervision are obligatory for therapists to attain needed competency before treating clients or conducting therapy research. Therefore, supervised training in EMDR therapy or any other evidence-based, trauma-informed treatment is essential for its ethical and effective application. We realize insisting that therapists and researchers obtain EMDR therapy training only from EMDR professional organizations has helped fuel an ongoing controversy, discussed in the next chapter. However, it is also acknowledged that, like all forms of psychotherapy, EMDR therapy is not a cure-all or panacea; not every client can be expected to have a positive outcome. Chapter 6 offers a glimpse into the potential future of EMDR research and therapy.

USE OF THIS BOOK

First and foremost, this monograph is not intended to be a substitute for EMDR therapy supervised training. We must emphasize that readers contemplating using EMDR therapy should receive appropriate training and supervision. We believe that this book can serve as a companion to the EMDR therapy textbook (F. Shapiro, 2018). Where possible, heavily redacted EMDR therapy transcripts are provided to help illustrate various constructs and treatment phases. In all cases, client confidentiality has been maintained.

EMDR THERAPY AND CULTURAL DIVERSITY

Mark Nickerson (2017d) highlighted the imperative of cultural competence in EMDR therapy. According to Nickerson (2017d), EMDR therapists can employ culturally informed adaptations to each of the eight phases as long as these modifications remain consistent with the AIP model and accomplish the goals of each phase. EMDR therapists are encouraged to develop cultural awareness so that they can adapt standard EMDR procedures to the cultural setting, build culturally sensitive therapeutic alliances, and take cultural aspects into consideration when implementing assessments, case formulations, and treatment plans. Hartung (2017) also described the importance of understanding cultural practices and customs when using EMDR in different professional societies in Asia, Europe, the Americas, and soon, in Africa, acknowledging the differing cultural concepts about mental health reflected in the history of mental health care in different countries.

Nickerson's (2017a) edited text includes research and adapted protocols for diverse and often marginalized populations, such as LGBTQ clients (e.g., Chang, 2017; O'Brien, 2017), Ugandan refugees (Masters et al., 2017), refugees and asylum seekers (Castelli Gattinara et al., 2017), clients dealing with ageism and classism (R. Shapiro, 2017), Latinx immigrants (Venkatraman & Siniego, 2017), and immigrant women (Lutz, 2017), as well as ways to explore and incorporate EMDR therapy in the healing of culturally based trauma and prejudice (Nickerson, 2017a, 2017b). In Chapter 5, we provide a sampling of EMDR research with African Americans and across the international community to include countries such as Africa, Germany, Indonesia, Iran, Sri Lanka, and Turkey.

2

History

The mind delights in a static environment that change from without . . .
seems in its very essence to be repulsive and an object of fear . . .
a little self-examination tells us pretty easily how deeply rooted
in the mind is the fear of the new.

—Wilfred Trotter, *Collected Papers*, discussing the response
by scientists to scientific discovery

In this chapter, we discuss the origins of eye movement desensitization and reprocessing (EMDR) therapy, its development, controversies, and its more recent history. Greater detail on the early days of EMDR and its growth is contained in *Eye Movement Desensitization and Reprocessing (EMDR) Therapy* (3rd ed.; F. Shapiro, 2018).

https://doi.org/10.1037/0000273-002
Eye Movement Desensitization and Reprocessing (EMDR) Therapy, by M. C. Russell and F. Shapiro

ORIGINS

The history of EMDR can be traced back to a series of serendipitous observations. In 1987, I (F. S.) was walking in a park while thinking about a highly anxiety-provoking event and noticed that my disturbing thoughts abruptly faded away without any conscious or deliberate attempt on my part. Curious, I purposely recalled the same event and noticed the bothersome thoughts were less vivid, and I was considerably less anxious. This was quite unexpected and surprising. Through introspection, I gradually came to realize a possible association between the diminishing emotional disturbance and spontaneous, rapid eye movements while walking (e.g., looking up and down, side-to-side). At that point, I started making deliberate eye movements while focusing on a number of disturbing memories and discovered that my negative reactions to these past events greatly lessened. Several days later, I began asking friends, colleagues, and others to think about a disturbing event from their past while simultaneously moving their eyes back and forth in a rapid manner. However, it soon became evident that the majority of people, including myself, could only sustain the eye movements for a short time. As an alternative to self-induced eye movements, I decided to start asking people to follow my fingers with their eyes as my hand made rapid left-to-right movements in a slightly diagonal direction. The vast majority of people similarly reported experiencing positive shifts in how they thought, remembered, and/or felt about their upsetting events. However, many people reported an interruption or blocking of the processing of their memories, so I began to experiment by using different speeds and directions of the eye movements, as well as asking people to focus on a different aspect of the memory (e.g., if they started with a disturbing thought, I would ask them to be aware of a feeling, a physical sensation in their body). Through this trial and error period involving some 70 people over a 6-month time frame, I developed a rudimentary protocol.

My theoretical orientation early in my career leaned toward behaviorism and the work of Joseph Wolpe, in particular, so I named the procedure eye movement desensitization (EMD). Initially, EMD was viewed as a counterconditioning treatment, grounded in behavioral-oriented theory, that used rapid eye movements from tracking the therapist's back and forth hand gestures to elicit desensitization. In 1987, EMD began to be tested empirically. Because the initial experience with EMD involved old or less distressing memories, it was decided to test EMD with individuals similarly bothered by past disturbing events. Consequently, the first candidates to formally receive EMD therapy were Vietnam War veterans and sexual molestation and rape survivors, all of whom experienced a Criterion A traumatic event required for a posttraumatic stress disorder (PTSD) diagnosis per the *Diagnostic and Statistical Manual of Mental Disorders* (3rd ed.; American Psychiatric Association, 1980).

Research participants were randomly assigned to either an EMD treatment group or a control group, where they were asked to describe their past trauma in detail without eye movements. Both groups were asked to identify a disturbing image of their traumatic event, along with negative beliefs or self-statements about the situation (e.g., I'm weak)—referred to as a negative cognition. Participants were then asked to rate the intensity of their anxiety along a 0–10 continuum or what Wolpe and Abrams (1991) referred to as the Subjective Units of Disturbance Scale, with 0 indicating the *absence of distress* and 10 representing *highest possible anxiety*. In addition, positive beliefs or self-statements about the traumatic event (e.g., I'm a survivor) were also assessed, referred to as positive cognition (PC). Participants rated how true their PC currently felt to them using a 7-point scale called the Validity of Cognition (VOC) scale, whereby 1 signified a *completely false* statement, and 7 indicated a *completely true* statement.

Within a single 90-minute session, the EMD treatment group reported a statistically significant desensitization effect characterized by a reduction in their anxiety or distress compared with the control group; they simultaneously reported significant cognitive restructuring, as indicated by an increase in their adaptive or positive self-statements (on the VOC) in contrast to the controls (F. Shapiro, 1989). At the end of the initial trial, participants in the control group also received EMD with similar reports of significant change. EMD treatment effects were maintained over a 1- and 3-month follow-up period. However, major limitations of the fledgling

EMD study included potential experimenter bias in that the researcher and treatment provider were one and the same, as well as the absence of standardized symptom measures and blind evaluations. The findings of the promising EMD clinical trials were published in 1989 by the *Journal of Traumatic Stress* (F. Shapiro, 1989).

That same year (1989), the Department of Veterans Affairs (DVA) published their first-ever randomized controlled trial (RCT) for PTSD, using the behavioral therapy method of prolonged imaginal exposure as inpatient treatment for Vietnam combat veterans, reporting moderate effects after six to 14 sessions (Cooper & Clum, 1989). The implications of a potentially more rapid, well-tolerated, and efficient treatment, particularly with regard to chronic PTSD, incited a great deal of excitement and appropriate skepticism both within and outside the DVA. To spur EMDR research and use in the DVA and Department of Defense (DoD), EMDR trainings were offered at no cost to any interested DVA and military therapists and researchers.

PARADIGM SHIFT

While attending graduate school in Palo Alto, California, I (M. C. R.) served as Francine Shapiro's research assistant at the Mental Research Institute from 1990–1991, assisting in the development of EMD theory. Consequently, in 1990, EMD was changed to EMDR to better account for a rapid, broader, more integrative information reprocessing effect versus a strict desensitization paradigm (F. Shapiro, 2018). Specifically, no extant behavioral or cognitive behavior theory appeared to adequately explain why EMDR worked by asking participants to momentarily recall a distressing event while visually tracking the therapists' left-to-right hand movements and encouraging free associations versus sustained exposure and preventing avoidance behaviors.

The EMDR name change reflected an abandonment of scientifically acceptable mainstream cognitive behavior theories of reciprocal inhibition and emotional processing in favor of an unproven but more integrative information processing–based paradigm initially referred to as the accelerated information processing model, which was later changed to the adaptive information processing (AIP) paradigm (see Chapter 3). In addition, in 1990, the EMDR Institute was founded and developed professional training standards. The shift in the theoretical paradigm and implementation of EMDR training standards intensified the controversy surrounding EMDR, especially as media reports of a single-session cure circulated.

THE EMDR CONTROVERSY

Since its 1989 introduction, the legitimacy of EMDR therapy has been the subject of a lengthy and impassioned scientific debate among EMDR advocates and critics. The ongoing decades-long controversy varies from personal attacks over the credentials of EMDR's founder and method of discovery to critiques over introducing a new psychotherapy theory that challenges the dominant cognitive behavior zeitgeist (Russell, 2008a), as well as a steady back and forth between researchers debating the quality of EMDR efficacy and dismantling research, along with accusations of proprietary EMDR professional organizations (Russell, 2008a).

EVIDENCE OF RESISTANCE TO EMDR BASED ON PROFESSIONAL STANDING

At least some measure of resistance to EMDR originates from the view that I (F. S.) lacked the scientific résumé to challenge the cognitive behavior therapy (CBT) zeitgeist. For instance, Carroll (n.d.) wrote, "The therapy was discovered by therapist Dr. Francine Shapiro, while on a walk in the park. . . . (Shapiro's doctorate was earned at a now defunct and never accredited Professional School of Psychological Studies)" (para. 3). EMDR therapy has also been derided by Harvard-trained DVA psychologist Richard McNally over how it was discovered: "Both Mesmer and Shapiro had their therapeutic epiphanies while walking outdoors" (McNally, 1999, p. 227).

EVIDENCE OF A THEORETICAL TURF WAR

In 1991, EMDR received an initial boost in credibility after the behavioral stalwart Joseph Wolpe published a case study of EMD, revealing its promise as a PTSD treatment (Wolpe & Abrams, 1991). At that time, the use of eye movements was hypothesized to represent merely a neutral or distracting stimulus that induced a relaxation response in a classic counter-conditioning paradigm. As long as EMD(R) proponents stayed within the lane of established behavioral constructs, scientific resistance would be minimal. However, the 1990 name change to EMDR and adoption of a novel yet unproven theoretical tenet exacerbated the controversy. For instance, leading EMDR critics openly admitted that "had EMDR been put forth simply as another variant of extant treatments, we suspect that much of the controversy over its efficacy and mechanism of action could have been avoided" (Lohr et al., 1999, p. 201). This sentiment was echoed by Terence Keane, the distinguished Veterans Affairs (VA) PTSD expert, who remarked, "The primary weakness of EMDR stems from a distinct lack of integration with existing models of psychopathology and psycho-therapy" (Keane, 1998, p. 404).

Today, EMDR therapy is often described as a CBT variant incorpo-rating exposure and cognitive restructuring (e.g., DVA & DoD, 2017). However, unlike trauma-focused talk therapies, EMDR does not require repetitive client reading or vivid retelling of their trauma narratives, nor is there any use of cognitive retraining or a requirement for hours of out-side homework (see Chapter 4). In fact, EMDR therapy requires therapists to follow clients' free associations to untargeted memories until clients report the absence of change. Only then are clients instructed to recall the initial traumatic memory. At best, EMDR represents sloppy exposure and cognitive therapy.

DEBATE OVER THE POTENTIALLY BIASED INTERPRETATION OF EMDR RESEARCH

Initial skepticism over EMDR's nontraditional methodology (i.e., use of eye movements) and reported single-session effects (F. Shapiro, 1989) was understandable and necessary, especially given the absence of subsequent RCTs to determine efficacy (Russell, 2008a). Multiple case studies by DVA researchers such as Howard Lipke, director of PTSD programs at the VA Medical Center, Great Lakes (e.g., Lipke & Botkin, 1992), eventually spurred RCTs. However, early EMDR-related RCTs were heavily critiqued on both sides of the debate on methodological grounds with evolving gold, revised gold, and platinum standards employed to analyze methodological rigor (Hertlein & Ricci, 2004).

CLINICAL PRACTICE GUIDELINE FOR THE MANAGEMENT OF POSTTRAUMATIC STRESS

In 2004, the DVA and DoD published the first U.S.-based clinical practice guidelines for the treatment of traumatic stress. After an extensive literature review, four Tier 1 evidence-based psychotherapies were identified as providing "significant benefit" for PTSD: cognitive therapy, exposure therapy, stress-inoculation training, and EMDR therapy. With regard to EMDR, the guideline reported the following:

- The possibility of obtaining significant clinical improvements in PTSD in a few sessions presents this treatment method [EMDR] as an attractive modality worthy of consideration (p. I-24).
- EMDR processing is internal to the patient, who does not have to reveal the traumatic event (p. I-24).

Amid a long and often acrimonious debate over EMDR theory, sufficient RCTs and meta-analyses eventually established the efficacy of EMDR according to nearly every other major domestic and international trauma guideline. For instance, the World Health Organization (WHO; 2013) recommended EMDR therapy as a "first line of treatment for post-traumatic stress disorder in adults" (p. 40) before prescribing selective serotonin reuptake inhibitors and tricyclic antidepressants. Specifically, WHO cited several key advantages of EMDR therapy in that it does not involve "(a) detailed descriptions of the traumatic event(s), (b) direct challenging of beliefs, (c) extended exposure, or (d) homework" (p. 1), resulting in its identification as a top-tier trauma-focused psychotherapy.

Despite widespread international recognition of EMDR as an efficacious trauma-based therapy, the controversy surrounding EMDR therapy research has persisted and is well-documented. For instance, the one notable exception to the worldwide recognition of EMDR as a top empirically supported psychotherapy is the practice guidelines from the American Psychological Association (APA; 2017a). The APA task force concluded that EMDR was only "conditionally" recommended due to the reported paucity of valid treatment outcomes. However, a detailed rebuttal indicated critical errors and inconsistencies in the statistical analysis of the strength of evidence, coupled with the inexplicable omission of several RCTs that every other major domestic and international practice guideline included in their meta-analyses, thus resulting in a downgrading of EMDR's evidence base (Dominguez & Lee, 2017).

SHIFTING THE DEBATE TO MECHANISM OF ACTION

With substantial empirical evidence now supporting EMDR therapy as an evidence-based, trauma-focused therapy, arguments have returned to earlier debates regarding its purported mechanism of action—namely, the efficacy of eye movements or other forms of bilateral stimulation. EMDR's theory has been labeled as pseudoscience (Herbert et al., 2000). In fact, some have argued that "given that the only active component of EMDR is already part of successful intervention for PTSD (e.g., CBT) it would seem more appropriate to focus research and training resources on improving these established interventions, rather than on EMDR" (Ost, 2006, p. 5). This viewpoint is echoed by a renowned VA researcher with the National Center of PTSD: "EMDR is distinguished from traditional desensitization treatment by its addition of induced eye movement to imaginal exposure, and if the defining element of EMDR is therapeutically inert, then there is little reason to investigate EMDR quo EMDR" (McNally, 1999, p. 3).

While the statement is accurate in that a meta-analysis of EMDR dismantling studies reported some studies not showing a robust treatment effect of eye movements (Bisson & Andrew, 2007), there have now been over 25 dismantling studies demonstrating positive effects for the eye-movement component used in EMDR therapy (see Chapter 5, this volume). Yet, even in 2020, mainstream organizations such as the National Center for PTSD appear to continue to undermine the status of EMDR research "Some research shows that the back-and-forth movements is an important part of treatment, but other research shows the opposite" (U. S. Department of Veterans Affairs, 2020, para. 2).

However, EMDR therapy is far from unique in having troubles finding empirical support for hypothesized treatment components; dismantling issues regarding CBT remain unresolved (e.g., Baskin et al., 2003). In fact, Alan Kazdin (2005) declared,

> Perhaps the most neglected question in therapy research is the mechanisms by which treatment leads to change. For even our most well-studied, evidence-based treatments (e.g., cognitive therapy for depression) we do not know why the treatment works (i.e., through what process). (p. 185)

We fully concur that more research is needed in terms of EMDR therapy's purported mechanisms of action; however, it is also worth noting that EMDR ought not to be singled out in this regard.

CRITICISM OVER EMDR THERAPY'S PROPRIETARY DISSEMINATION

In 1993, randomized EMDR trials began with varying levels of improvement from little to none (Jensen, 1994) to modest (Boudewyns & Hyer, 1996; Pitman et al., 1996; Rogers et al., 1999) to significant (Carlson et al., 1998; Silver et al., 1995). A subsequent meta-analysis revealed significant associations between EMDR treatment fidelity and treatment effect sizes (Maxfield & Hyer, 2002).

Critiques of researchers employing EMDR without sufficient fidelity to the standard protocol led to rebuttals and calls that researchers undergo appropriate EMDR training. At that time, it was common for behavioral and CBT therapists and researchers to rely on self-training by reading published clinical works of a particular modality or new CBT variant. The situation became increasingly tense when the only formal EMDR training was being offered by EMDR professional organizations, resulting in allegations of proprietary practice. However, it was also not uncommon for certain therapeutic approaches to strongly advocate for formal training such as psychoanalysis and biofeedback.

In 1990, the EMDR Institute was founded to offer standardized training in EMDR therapy for therapists and researchers. To address issues regarding treatment fidelity and client safety, I (F. S.) organized a two-part EMD training that included supervised practicums by therapists who served as EMDR facilitators after being trained by me. The initial EMD training consisted of a 1.5-day Part 1 basic training. Afterward, trainees were expected to practice EMD(R) and subsequently attend a 1-day advanced training. Around the same time, I began to receive troubling reports of clients being harmed by recently trained EMDR therapists who had started training others. Consequently, EMDR trainees were required to sign written agreements to not teach EMDR until they were deemed qualified. The training restrictions were lifted with the publication of the EMDR textbook (F. Shapiro, 1995). However, the requirement that researchers and therapists alike attend sanctioned EMDR training to avoid future criticism concerning possible negative findings, along with my prohibition against trainees from teaching EMDR, added fuel to the criticisms of proprietary practice (i.e., Herbert et al., 2000).

In 1995, the EMDR International Association (EMDRIA; https://www.emdria.org) was founded to establish international standards for training, certification, and practice, and I published the first EMDR textbook: *Eye Movement Desensitization and Reprocessing: Basic Principles, Protocols, and Procedures* (F. Shapiro, 1995). EMDR training increasingly became longer and more expensive. At present, the two-part EMDR training is now 3 days for each part and taught only by EMDR Institute– or EMDRIA-approved trainers and facilitators. Part 1 trainees are required to complete at least 10 hours of consultation with an EMDRIA-approved consultant before attending the second part of training. Certified EMDR therapists, trainers, facilitators, and consultants are all required to complete a certain number of annual EMDR continuing education credits taught by sanctioned EMDR organizational members.

In short, we are split on the merits of accusations about the proprietary dissemination of EMDR therapy. I (F. S.) insist that EMDR training standards ensure quality control, client safety, and the continuing education of clinicians. However, I (M. C. R.) believe an objective appraisal of EMDR dissemination warrants such criticism. For instance, I (M. C. R.) am unaware of any empirical support for the ever-expanding training length and certification requirements. However, there is evidence to the contrary.

In 1995, the Coatesville, Pennsylvania VA Medical Center PTSD program director, Dr. Steven M. Silver, a naval flight officer in the Vietnam War, provided the first of many EMDR trainings to DVA therapists. Furthermore, in response to the 1995 Oklahoma City bombing, an FBI agent who had previously received EMDR therapy called the EMDR Institute to request help, stating that local mental health professionals were overwhelmed by the task. Consequently, the EMDR Humanitarian Assistance Program (HAP) was established to focus on building the capacity of underserved domestic and international communities, secure effective trauma treatment through proper training, and develop local Trauma Recovery Network chapters.

In 2006, I (M. C. R.) became the first active-duty U.S. military EMDR trainer to conduct a series of joint DoD and DVA regional EMDR trainings with Dr. Silver and other DVA trainers (Russell et al., 2007). The trainings were sponsored by EMDR HAP. Given the hectic schedules of military mental health professionals during a time of war, the EMDR HAP trainings were significantly condensed from 6-day to two all-day trainings, combining both basic and advanced curriculum from standard EMDRIA-approved training. The EMDR trainers went into five different regions and offered free EMDR training to 175 active-duty mental health providers, civilian contractors, and DVA clinicians (Russell et al., 2007). Trainees receiving the abbreviated EMDR training voluntarily submitted results of chart reviews conducted at their sites when implementing the

EMDR training. EMDR baseline and PTSD symptom measures were obtained from 72 active-duty clients diagnosed with PTSD after receiving EMDR therapy (Russell et al., 2007). Results revealed significant improvement on all pre–post measures after an average of four EMDR therapy sessions, eight if the client was wounded in action. Although clear methodological limitations exist, this study was the first to demonstrate EMDR training efficacy.

WHAT IS THE POTENTIAL HARM TODAY FROM PERPETUATING THE EMDR CONTROVERSY?

In 1998, a rigorous RCT was conducted by the DVA with Vietnam War combat veterans diagnosed with PTSD, resulting in 77% of veterans losing the PTSD diagnosis after 12 therapy sessions (Carlson et al., 1998), which marked the last EMDR RCT by the VA. Since 2001, the American (and other) militaries have been involved in the Afghanistan and Iraq Wars. Yet despite the steady drumbeat of skyrocketing PTSD and suicide rates amongst veterans and the fact that EMDR has earned a top-tier recommendation in its clinical practice guidelines (DVA & DoD, 2004, 2017), EMDR research has inexplicably been shunned by the DVA since 1998. Moreover, the DoD has conducted RCTs involving acupuncture, yoga, MDMA, and a host of other unproven treatments but has failed to conduct a single EMDR trial during the past 20 years of war. Why is that?

In 2007, the Institute of Medicine (IOM) was commissioned by the DVA to reassess PTSD treatments, resulting in the first review to conclude there was insufficient evidence of EMDR therapy's efficacy (IOM, 2007). The explanation offered by the IOM (2007) was that there was a paucity of quality RCTs for treating combat-related PTSD. However, the IOM (2007) failed to acknowledge its circular reasoning in that the very agencies responsible for researching EMDR (DVA and DoD) have neglected their obligations. Not surprisingly, a pointed rebuttal was published contradicting the IOM's (2007) analysis of existent RCTs it excluded (Lee & Schubert, 2009), thus adding fuel to the flames of controversy.

There is no explanation or justification for perpetuating a controversy that harms veterans, their families, and greater society. A further example of today's harm caused by scientific bias is that the last National Institute of Mental Health (NIMH) funded EMDR trial was conducted by Bessel van der Kolk et al. (2007). Van der Kolk et al. conducted a double-blind, placebo-controlled RCT that found EMDR to be superior to Prozac and a wait-list condition for both adult-onset PTSD and adults with child-onset PTSD (van der Kolk et al., 2007).

The most recent back-and-forth debate about the status of EMDR treatment research lends credibility to claims that the 32-year-old controversy surrounding EMDR is largely a consequence of it posing a direct challenge to the mainstream CBT and psychopharmacological zeitgeists (e.g., Russell, 2008a). Maladaptive resistance to properly researched EMDR therapy by such vaunted institutions as the DoD, IOM, NIMH, and DVA harms current and future clients and serves as an unnecessary, self-inflicted impediment for future discoveries of effective psychotherapy.

While the United States is mired in a self-manufactured controversy over EMDR therapy, the rest of the international community has moved forward (e.g., WHO, 2013).

3

Theory

The theoretical basis and treatment principles of eye movement desensitization and reprocessing (EMDR) are based on the adaptive information processing (AIP) theory that also provides an explanation for the origin of psychopathology and personality development (F. Shapiro, 2018). In short, the AIP model of EMDR is an integrative neuropsychological approach positing that associative or neural memory networks form the physiological bases of perception, cognition, emotion, and behavior in health and pathology. Neural (memory) networks are composed of past experiences that are physically stored as multiple components encoded at the time, involving sensory stimuli (i.e., images, sounds, pain, smells, tastes), emotions, thoughts or beliefs, somatic sensations, and/or behavioral reactions. For example, if a client is involved in a major earthquake, they may report seeing their house swaying and objects falling off the shelves, coupled with a loud rumbling noise, accompanied

https://doi.org/10.1037/0000273-003
Eye Movement Desensitization and Reprocessing (EMDR) Therapy, by M. C. Russell and F. Shapiro

by feelings of fear with the physical sensations of heart pounding, profuse sweating, and trembling, along with the thought "I'm going to die!" and behaviorally yelling for their pet dog as they run to take cover under the kitchen table (see Figure 3.1).

The nature of our memory networks is that the earthquake memory now becomes associated or linked up to similar life experiences, whether it was prior earthquake exposures or other earlier potentially life-threatening events when the client felt terrified, hopeless, or helpless or thought they might die.

THREE FUNDAMENTAL PRINCIPLES OF THE AIP MODEL

The AIP model consists of three core principles essential for understanding EMDR therapy.

Principle 1: The Intrinsic Information Processing System

The first principle is that the brain has evolved an intrinsic information processing capacity that enables human beings to reorganize their reactions to disturbing life events from an initial dysfunctional state of disequilibrium to a state of adaptive resolution. According to the AIP model, the brain's inherent information processing systems, like other bodily systems, are physiologically geared toward healthy adaptation to aid survival. For example, the body reflexively heals a physical wound or cut unless something inhibits the natural healing process and an infection ensues. Similarly, our digestive system is designed to extract adaptive elements needed to survive and eliminate the rest. We reasoned that it made sense that our neurological system similarly functions to extract necessary and adaptive information from our life experiences while eliminating the remainder.

When healthy people are exposed to distressing events such as being publicly chastised by a teacher, parent, or work supervisor, it is normal to initially experience a stress response that may involve increased heart rate, elevated blood pressure, irrational thoughts including self-blame,

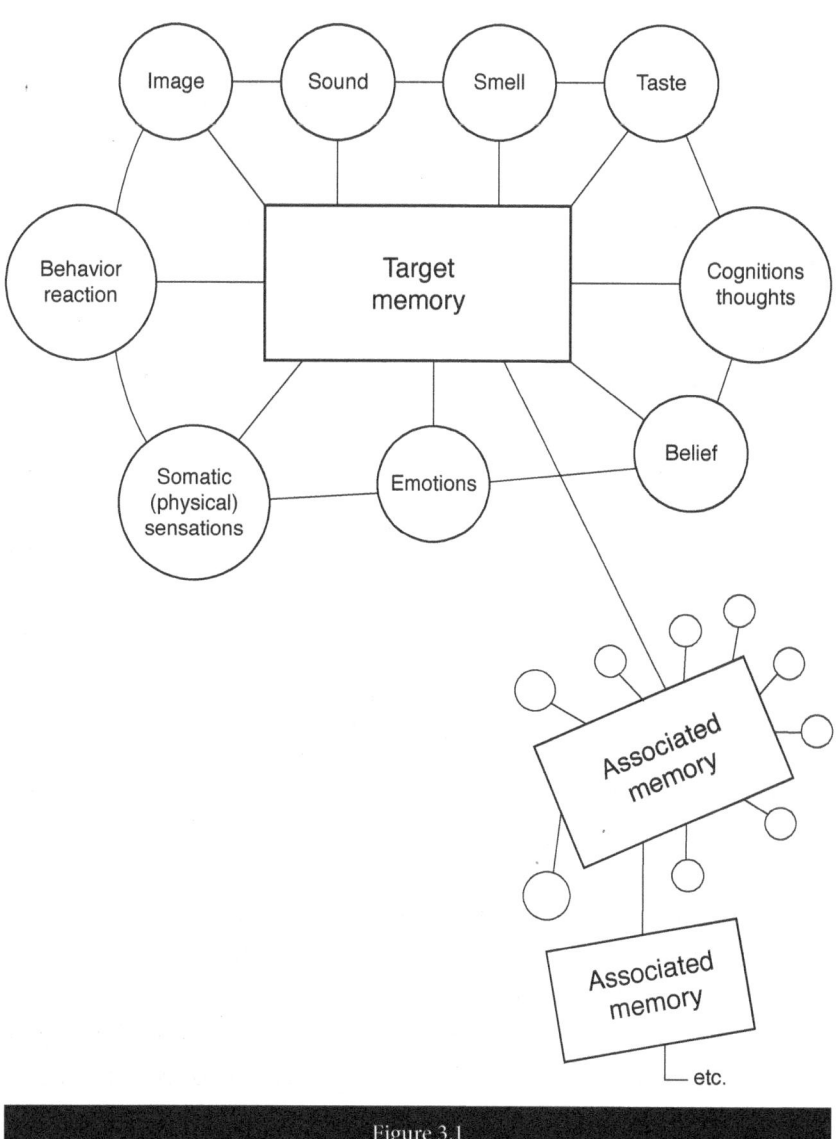

Figure 3.1

Neural (memory) networks.

or a behavioral impulse to fight, flee, or freeze. Afterward, the person may think about the event and possibly even ruminate or worry. They may feel angry, embarrassed, or ashamed. They may talk to friends, family, or trusted coworkers; go on a walk; or write an email or text to a confidant. They may dream about it and try to ascertain what could be learned from the experience. Was the chastiser just having a bad day, or are they habitually a jerk? Is there something the targeted person had done or failed to do? The memory of being publicly scorned becomes associated or linked to similar negative life experiences. Over a brief period, the healthy person resolves their distress and learns from the experience. As they do so, their physiological systems return to a state of balance or homeostasis. Their cognitive and emotional perspectives are also adaptive (e.g., "I'm okay") as they imagine and rehearse assertively confronting the chastiser privately. The next day, the person appropriately talks to the offending individual, and the chastiser rightly apologizes for their insensitive behavior. This memory becomes linked to earlier positive experiences of mastery that helped us adapt and survive.

Principle 2: Chronic or Potentially Traumatic Stressors Can Block Adaptive Processing

The second principle of the AIP model posits that chronic stress and potentially traumatic events, especially during developmental life phases, can interfere or block the brain's information processing system. In other words, traumatic or other highly emotionally charged events can overwhelm the brain's capacity to assimilate or accommodate information, which can become stored as unprocessed experiences in maladaptive memory networks. Psychopathological symptoms and conditions, therefore, represent the activation of these maladaptive neural networks, resulting in selective attention and conditional responses to negative current stimuli and experiences, as well as anticipating future threats, loss, and pain.

As a consequence of disrupting emotional information processing due to excess arousal from trauma and/or chronic distress, the information related to the stressors is often stored in a state-specific, dysfunctional form that fails to reach an adaptive resolution. There is evidence that traumatic memories are stored in an implicit, short-term memory system that contains sensory impressions and emotional and somatic reactions (Stickgold, 2002). Our earliest memories of attachment and other life events during the formative years serve as foundational experiences for interpreting and making meaning of our current experiences. External and internal stimuli trigger reactions, which may or may not be conscious but are evidence of the activation of memory networks.

Principle 3: Bilateral Stimulation Activates the Brain's Intrinsic Information Processing System

The third AIP model principle purports that *bilateral stimulation*, defined as rapid, alternating (left-to-right) eye movements, sounds, or kinesthetic vibrations, serves to mimic or activate the brain's intrinsic information processing system processing disturbing events and dysfunctionally stored memories toward an adaptive resolution. According to Leeds (2009),

> Central to this third principle is the concept of self-healing, which is analogous to what occurs with physical injuries. Surgeons can remove blockages to healing such as foreign objects or tumors, and create conditions favorable to healing but then they must "let nature take its course." No surgeon can make a wound heal. Only the body itself can do that. This capacity is encoded in our DNA and expressed through the innate reparative systems of the body. (p. 22)

In the case of traumatic stress or other psychological injuries, the AIP model posits that the client's experiences are often stored in an unprocessed, state-specific form (as if the event is happening now) and that the therapist cannot directly heal the person. At best, the therapist creates the necessary conditions for healing. In EMDR therapy, that involves using dual-focused attention and bilateral stimulation in the context of the eight EMDR treatment phases and therapeutic alliance. In other words, the EMDR therapist must learn to trust the brain–body's natural healing processes.

PSYCHOPATHOLOGY AND RESILIENCE

In the AIP model, most types of psychopathology reflect dysfunctionally stored and/or unprocessed or unintegrated information in neural networks that influences and is triggered by present experiences and anticipated future events (e.g., repeatedly envisioning worst-case scenarios). The particular brain circuits involved and consequent pattern or combination of physical and psychological symptoms presented give rise to different diagnostic classifications (e.g., posttraumatic stress disorder [PTSD], depression, substance abuse, somatization). However, the etiology, maintenance, and/or exacerbation of most pathological states is believed to be due to the underlying, unprocessed components of disturbing or traumatic experiences. We consider early pivotal incidents that establish dysfunctional affects, beliefs, somatic symptoms, and behaviors as *touchstone events*, and these are regularly targeted in EMDR therapy, along with other memories associatively linked in a dysfunctional memory network. Like cognitive information processing models (i.e., Beck's cognitive therapy), AIP asserts that the more expansive or active a dysfunctional network, the greater propensity for selective attention and distorted interpretations and reactions to current and future stimuli, a phenomenon that maintains maladaptive behavior.

Pathologic or maladaptive patterns of behavior signify that the brain's natural self-healing or processing mechanism is blocked. Unlike the majority of life experiences that often include adversity, certain highly distressful, emotionally charged, or traumatic events may not readily be assimilated or accommodated and thus may not be properly processed, integrated, and stored in an adaptive memory network. Therefore, identifying and targeting past, present, and future (anticipated) pathogenic experiential contributors—whether conventional *DSM* Criterion A or big "T" traumatic events (i.e., combat) or less conventional, yet equally disturbing (small "t") traumatic experiences (e.g., unwanted divorce)— is essential for adaptive processing or healing to occur (F. Shapiro, 2018). EMDR is used to address the underlying experiences that contribute to clinical problems and health by using the three-pronged approach giving attention to the past, present, and future.

Resilience and posttraumatic growth are readily observable in EMDR therapy. Per the AIP model, the adaptive neural networks register our positive attachments, resilience, coping resources, and sense of efficacy, while maladaptive networks emerge with repeated experiences of adverse life events; negative attachment; vulnerability; inescapable fear, pain, and loss; and personal failures. Clients often spontaneously generate their own adaptive appraisals as they gain access to their adaptive memory networks. For instance, I (M. C. R.) treated an adult client who suffered a traumatic leg amputation after a motorcycle accident (Russell, 2008b). In addition to being diagnosed with PTSD and major depressive disorder, the client complained of an array of phantom limb pain and sensations. His overriding negative belief "I'm weak" caused the client considerable shame when seen in public walking on crutches with a single leg. During a set of bilateral stimulation (eye movements), the client was processing the phantom limb sensations when suddenly his facial expression and posture changed. He smiled and altered his position from slouching to sitting up straight. After the eye movements, he was asked, "What are you noticing now?" The client responded, "I was just remembering something I hadn't thought about in a very long time. . . . My father owned a steel company, and the motto of his company was 'Jones's steel bends but doesn't break!'"

The client was instructed to "stay with that, Jones's steel bends but doesn't break, and notice the phantom limb pain in your leg," which was followed by additional eye movements. During the eye movements, the client continued to be transformed into a state of "strength." The client accessed his adaptive memory network that was now being linked to the traumatic event and phantom limb. From that point forward, the client's cognitions rapidly shifted in a more adaptive manner. He no longer feared going out in public or feeling ashamed or weak—in fact, just the opposite. The final positive cognition he adopted was "I am strong." This change in self-appraisal translated into a significant reduction in psychological symptoms and phantom limb sensations (Russell, 2008b).

HYPOTHESIZED MECHANISMS OF ACTION

Over the past decade, research has investigated various mechanisms of action. Multiple mechanisms may be activated during EMDR therapy to produce the accelerated treatment effects. According to the AIP model, EMDR treatment effects are the result of essentially two key components: (a) dual-focused attention and (b) bilateral stimulation in the context of a safe, effective therapeutic alliance.

Dual-Focused Attention

Dual-focused attention occurs when clients are asked to divide their attention between internal stimuli and rapidly alternating external stimuli (i.e., a distressing image, thought, emotion, or sensation), thereby accessing the dysfunctional memory network while simultaneously attending to rapidly alternating (left–right) rhythmic external stimuli (i.e., eye movements, auditory tones, kinesthetic vibrations). This dual focus strikes a balance with the often-problematic extremes of excessive self-focused attention (or self-absorption), whereby individuals are prone to excluding external information and the equally dysfunctional state of extreme hypervigilance or externally focused attention for anticipated threats and/or avoidance of internal stimuli (i.e., emotions). For instance, negative attentional bias has long been associated with PTSD, and EMDR therapy was found to reduce attentional biases linked to PTSD symptom reduction (El Khoury-Malhame et al., 2011; Pineles et al., 2009). Physiological correlates of dual-attention tasks and EMDR therapy have been reviewed by Schubert and colleagues (2011).

A recent meta-analysis by Houben and colleagues (2020) examined 15 randomized controlled trials (RCTs) involving 942 participants and found that eye movements combined with dual-focused attention resulted in a significant decrease in the vividness and emotional distress associated with target memories. In another study, Lee et al. (2006) examined the responses of 44 clients receiving EMDR therapy for PTSD. An independent rater was used to assess the level of detached attentional focus and found that the greatest reduction of PTSD symptoms coincided with the client processing their traumatic memories in a more detached manner (Lee et al., 2006), which is consistent with our hypothesis of the role of dual-focused attention (F. Shapiro, 2018). Similarly, behavioral researchers found that the splitting of participant's attentional focus via dual tasking significantly reduced fear conditioning (Leer et al., 2013).

Bilateral Stimulation

Much of the recent controversy around EMDR revolves around disputes about whether eye movements or other bilateral stimulation forms are essential or inert components. For instance, Hyer and Brandsma (1997) asserted that EMDR is basically good exposure therapy without the eye movements.

The term *bilateral stimulation* (BLS) refers to the fact that sensory and motor pathways are lateralized. For example, most of the optic and motor nerve pathways from the right eye cross over and are processed by the left visual cortex and vice versa. Therefore, the physical movements of one's eyes from left to right in EMDR activates both brain hemispheres (Lee et al., 2019). Jeffries and Davis (2013) conducted a review of the research on eye movements in EMDR, concluding that eye movements are a critical component responsible for EMDR's treatment effects.

Similarly, auditory and kinesthetic stimuli alternatively presented to the left and right sides activate both cerebral hemispheres. Lateralization also refers to the fact that each cerebral hemisphere is lateralized or specializes in processing certain kinds of information. For instance, it has been shown that negative valence emotions (i.e., fear, anxiety, anger) tend to be processed more by the right hemisphere and positive emotions (i.e., joy, contentment) by the left hemisphere. Interestingly, functional brain imaging studies of clients successfully treated for PTSD with EMDR reveal significant pre–post changes in brain function and lateralization effects, whereby previously overactive right-hemispheric circuits (i.e., amygdala) and hypoactive, typically left prefrontal circuits are reversed and correspond with clinically significant self-reported changes in PTSD symptoms. For instance, using functional magnetic resonance imaging (fMRI), EMDR therapy was found to be linked with increased activity in the left hippocampus and left amygdala (Rousseau, El Khoury-Malhame, Reynaud, Boukezzi, et al., 2019). Rousseau and colleagues (2020) used fMRI to examine what occurs during auditory BLS and without BLS and found that auditory BLS results in significant activation of large emotional neural networks, thus giving credence to the idea that alternate forms of BLS can be successfully applied.

Additional neuroimaging studies have reported an increase in hippocampal volume in patients undergoing EMDR therapy for PTSD (Bossini et al., 2017), as well as left amygdala volumetric increase (e.g., Laugharne et al., 2016), increased prefrontal cortex gray matter (Boukezzi et al., 2017), and functional normalization in limbic structures associated with PTSD (Lansing et al., 2005; Oh & Choi, 2004; Pagani et al., 2007, 2012).

To date, a meta-analysis (Lee & Cuijpers, 2013) and more than 30 RCTs have demonstrated that eye movements used in EMDR therapy are a significant determinant in positive clinical outcomes. It is currently hypothesized that BLS during EMDR therapy—namely, eye movements—produces accelerated information processing effects by (a) taxing working memory by engaging in two tasks (recall and eye movements; e.g., Baddeley, 2012; Thomaes et al., 2016); (b) stimulating the orienting response and its associated parasympathetic, relaxation response (e.g., M. M. Bradley, 2009; Landin-Romero et al., 2013); and (c) eliciting the same or similar emotional processing mechanism involved in rapid eye movement sleep (e.g., Elofsson et al., 2008; Pagaini et al., 2007; Stickgold, 2002). At present, the aforementioned hypotheses seem to align with our understanding of the neurobiology of memory reconsolidation, whereby recalling a memory can be associated with novel or existing adaptive information and then restored in a changed form (e.g., Suzuki et al., 2004). Presenting a distracting stimulus during the reactivation of a memory can interfere with its reconsolidation.

A number of neurophysiological studies provide evidence that successful EMDR therapy results in changes to the structure and functioning of brain areas involved in the facilitation of information processing and integration of memories (e.g., Landin-Romero et al., 2013). Van Veen and colleagues (2020) found that adding eye movements during imaginal exposure results in short-lived memory effects compared with exposure alone. In sum, despite the aforementioned, we fully acknowledge the need for greater research into the underlying mechanisms of EMDR therapy.

IS EXPOSURE THE MECHANISM OF ACTION?

The elicitation of dual-focused attention involves asking the client to recall and attend to a particular distressing memory and then introduces BLS. Afterward, EMDR incorporates a free-associative process that allows the relevant connections to be made by the client as they arise, with the EMDR therapist facilitating further dual-focus attention and BLS. These associations are often memories of events that have no obvious relevance to the targeted trauma, with the therapist not redirecting the client's attention back to the targeted experience until the end of the session. While asking a client to recall an event is a form of exposure, the aforementioned process is nearly 180 degrees opposite to exposure-based therapies that emphasize repetitive exposure to the target with avoidance prevention.

FORGING ADAPTIVE ASSOCIATIONS OF NEURAL NETWORKS

Reprocessing or learning is viewed as the forging or strengthening of adaptive associations between the maladaptive neural networks related to psychopathological states and adaptive neural networks that contain memories related to secure attachment, coping, mastery, self-efficacy, "lessons learned," and other "positive" or adaptive experiences stored in the brain. EMDR incorporates an associative memory process whereby perceptions of present stimuli or events are interpreted and responded to by linkage with neural networks containing similar experiences such as emotions, physical sensations, and thoughts and beliefs. Accessing the experience by directing self-focused attention to a memory creates a link between consciousness and where the information is stored. By-products of reprocessing include desensitization (decrease in disturbance) but also adaptive restructuring of the client's narrative, self-initiated insights, and perspectives, as well as changes in physical and emotional responses. Conceptually, this tendency of humans to process information to adaptive resolution is also consistent with basic assumptions of humanistic psychology (e.g., F. Shapiro, 2018).

WHY THEORY MATTERS

It is our most fervent belief and collective experience that to use EMDR effectively, the clinician must achieve a good understanding of the theoretical model because it informs most treatment choice points (i.e., when to return to the target memory), which can be the critical variable between a successful or unsuccessful outcome. In short, the clinician should remember that the EMDR therapist's functions are to (a) *access* the necessary memory networks by eliciting appropriate dual-focused attention in the context of a secure, therapeutic alliance; (b) *stimulate* the information processing system by maintaining dual focus attention and BLS in the presence of an attuned therapist; (c) *move* the information along the associative links of neural networks until adaptive resolution is achieved for past, present, and future experiential contributors; and (d) *reassess* the adaptive resolution of targeted memory networks (F. Shapiro, 2018).

COMPARATIVE THEORETICAL APPROACHES

EMDR can be described as an "integrative" psychotherapy for several reasons (F. Shapiro, 2018). First, and perhaps foremost, the clinician using EMDR will quickly recognize that many aspects from a diverse range of theoretical orientations will spontaneously emerge during the course of therapy (i.e., recall of early nonconscious memories, adaptive insights, client-generated solutions, cognitive restructuring, desensitization, somatic expression of pathology and health).

For the AIP model, (a) memory networks are the basis of perception, attitude, and behavior, and problems are the result of incompletely processed experiences; and (b) change is the result of forging associations between networks of information stored in the brain.

In the cognitive model, (a) cognitive distortion and faulty beliefs are the bases of maladaptive schemas or pathology; and (b) cognitions are changed through reframing, self-monitoring, and homework exercises.

For the behavioral model, (a) maladaptive behavior occurs as the result of faulty learning in the environment; and (b) behavior is changed through conditioning, exposure, modeling, and altering reinforcement patterns.

For the cognitive behavior model, (a) psychological dysfunction is understood in terms of mechanisms of learning and information processing, and (b) change is through a combination of behavioral and cognitive strategies.

In the psychodynamic model, (a) pathology results from unresolved, often early childhood experiences; and (b) change results from achieving insight into previously unconscious dynamics.

In the humanistic model, (a) pathology is viewed as a false, incongruous self, stunting personal growth; and (b) facilitating conditions for client-centered change in self and growth are necessary.

For the Gestalt model, (a) pathology is often represented by repressed, unfinished conflicts that are stored in the body; and (b) change occurs by releasing physiological expression of unfinished business.

In the neurobiological model, (a) pathology caused by alterations in neuroendocrine and hormonal dysregulation (i.e., through the hypothalamic–pituitary–adrenal axis) alters brain structure and functioning of memory, emotional, and executive control circuits; and (b) change occurs by resetting physiological and cerebral regulatory and information processing systems.

THE THERAPEUTIC RELATIONSHIP IN EMDR THERAPY

Some readers might come away with the impression that all an EMDR therapist essentially does is sit silently while waving their hand back and forth in front of the client's face. Others may think they will simply add eye movements to their standard practice of talk therapy, including ample paraphrasing, reflective statements, and other forms of active listening, or engage in the rational disputation of the client's faulty cognitions, inquire about the client's meaning making, or offer interpretations of the client's patterns. Neither viewpoint is accurate. The EMDR therapist is not a robot simulating windshield wipers, nor are they engaging in talk therapy.

As in all forms of psychotherapy, particularly trauma-focused treatments such as EMDR therapy, it is essential that the therapist establish a mutual sense of trust and supportive working alliance to be effective. In EMDR therapy, the therapist does not need to know all the details about the trauma, the client's thoughts and feelings, or the meanings of their self-statements. The EMDR therapist only needs to know from the client whether the information is shifting or changing and moving toward an adaptive resolution. The client is instructed to disclose to the therapist whatever they are comfortable disclosing. The EMDR therapist often has to check themselves against the frequent use of active listening or cognitive techniques, and instead, they must learn to trust the AIP model and structure of EMDR therapy. The EMDR therapist acts as a facilitator of change much as in person-centered approaches; however, there is also a directive component that is different from Rogerian therapy. Namely, the EMDR therapist must minimize their verbalizations and restart BLS as much as practicable.

When clients access highly emotionally charged material or abreaction, the EMDR therapist typically increases the frequency of supportive comments and encourages the client to continue with dual-focused attention and BLS. The reader is referred to F. Shapiro's 2018 textbook for a more detailed description of the AIP model and investigations of the theoretical constructs.

CULTURAL DIVERSITY AND THE AIP MODEL

The AIP model, along with the standard EMDR therapy eight-phases and three-pronged protocol, applies to all forms of traumatic experiences, including culturally based trauma (Nickerson, 2017c). According to Nickerson (2017d),

> From the AIP perspective, we want to understand our client's adaptive tendencies. We may wonder, "What is adaptive and what is

> maladaptive in the realm of social behavior?" "How is the formation of culture adaptive or maladaptive?" and most importantly, "How can we assist our clients to adapt to challenges and opportunities?" (p. 19)

The adverse impact of culturally experienced discrimination, prejudice, oppression, and stigma contains the characteristics of other traumatic assaults on the self. These experiences result in state-based memories that often influence an individual's sense of self, perceptions, and general welfare (Nickerson, 2017d). Ultimately, unresolved culturally based traumatic memories can be easily triggered and negatively impact an individual's development, sense of safety, identity, and sense of agency, as well as determine how people view and treat themselves and others (Nickerson, 2017b). Consequently, the past experiential contributors of racism, sexism, homophobia, ageism, ableism, and other isms should be considered as target memories in EMDR therapy, along with the triggering antecedents, future worries, and desired outcome.

4

The Therapy Process

I n this chapter, we examine the standard eye movement desensitization and reprocessing (EMDR) protocol. We provide considerable details about what each phase entails and how the EMDR therapist navigates within and between each phase. However, the chapter should not be construed as a substitute for supervised EMDR training. EMDR therapy is an eight-phase approach that seeks to address the full range of clinical symptoms caused or exacerbated by past adverse experiences. The initial phases include client history and preparation, followed by four reprocessing phases (assessment, desensitization, installation, body scan) where bilateral stimulation (BLS) is used. The last two phases are for ending and reinitiating EMDR treatment sessions (closure and reevaluation). A summary of the EMDR treatment phases can also be found in Appendix A. The following is an overview of the main goals and procedural objectives of the eight phases of EMDR therapy.

https://doi.org/10.1037/0000273-004
Eye Movement Desensitization and Reprocessing (EMDR) Therapy, by M. C. Russell and F. Shapiro

PHASE 1: CLIENT HISTORY

Phase 1 involves gathering information about the client's readiness for EMDR therapy, including identifying treatment goals, screening for suitability for trauma-focused work, assessing client strengths and coping "resources," and obtaining sufficient history to develop a comprehensive treatment plan (F. Shapiro, 2018). History taking examines many factors essential to ensure the client can safely be treated with EMDR at a given time, such as their premorbid level of functioning before the identified trauma, complexity of clinical presentations (comorbidity, quality of childhood experiences, attachments, and extent of trauma history), and current stability of their environment (Russell & Figley, 2013).

Client Safety and Suitability for Reprocessing

As in any trauma-focused work, therapists make a concerted effort to assess the client's readiness for EMDR processing. A detailed client history is critical for the therapist to become sufficiently informed about the client's possible experiences with EMDR processing both during and after treatment sessions. Accessing and stimulating information contained in the target memory will bring to consciousness those various memory components stored at the time of the event (e.g., emotions, physical sensations, sensory stimuli, dissociation) that can be disturbing for the client. Therefore, the therapist needs to properly assess the client's readiness and capacity to cope with the resurfacing of distressing information, as well as their responsiveness to guidance by the therapist during reprocessing; otherwise, extended preparation is required before any processing may ensue.

Decades of experience with EMDR teach us that even if the target memory seems relatively minor, it may rapidly transform to an intensely emotionally charged experience or link to a different but powerful experience. The core feature of EMDR is accelerated reprocessing with the possibility of the swift resurfacing of highly disturbing experiences; therefore, evaluating client readiness is critical. It is impossible to predict precisely how a client will respond to processing a targeted memory. Determining client suitability for EMDR is essentially no different than with other trauma-focused treatments. There are no unique contraindications specific to EMDR, except perhaps when using eye movements with someone with a history of retinal detachment or other current eye discomfort (F. Shapiro, 2018). Research has demonstrated EMDR to be effective with alternative BLS such as sounds, taps, or vibration pads held in the hands (i.e., Rousseau et al., 2020).

Possible Contraindication for EMDR Therapy

EMDR therapy reprocessing should be postponed when any of the following is present.

- *therapeutic alliance issues*: Trauma-focused work requires the client to feel comfortable with experiencing vulnerability, lack of control, and somatic symptoms when accessing the targeted memory. Although detailed self-disclosure is not required in EMDR, there must be sufficient trust and rapport for clients to truthfully report what they are experiencing. Clients with complex developmental trauma often have difficulty with trust and safety, requiring the therapist to properly prepare the client before proceeding to reprocessing during the client preparation phase. Specific EMDR treatment considerations and protocols adapted for working with children and adolescents are available (Adler-Tapia & Settle, 2016; Gomez, 2013). In situations in which adequate trust and rapport have not been established, EMDR therapy should not proceed.
- *timing issues*: If an imminent work, personal, or family crisis or urgent matter emerges that requires the client's full attention, postpone reprocessing until the crisis is resolved, when possible. Similarly, if the client and/or therapist will be taking a scheduled vacation or extended business trip, postpone starting EMDR therapy.
- *an imminent pending dangerous mission*: Military personnel, law enforcement, and other first responders who will be participating in an imminent (within 6 hours) high-risk activity as a result of their vocation should postpone EMDR therapy reprocessing until after the completion of the mission, when possible (Russell & Figley, 2013). Common

aftereffects of intense EMDR therapy reprocessing include fatigue and possible distractibility from continued internal reprocessing that may interfere with decision making and reaction time. Using the resource development and installation (RDI) protocol or other performance improvement strategies may be considered (Russell & Figley, 2013).

- *poor affect tolerance*: Clients presenting as emotionally unstable, with protracted periods of intense crying, anger, terror, or shame during client history taking may benefit from expanded preparation exercises such as RDI or related procedures to develop affective tolerance and regulation skills before EMDR therapy reprocessing (see Phase 2). That said, it is strongly recommended that the therapist introduce a self-control technique such as the safe and calm place exercise to assess possible suitability for EMDR (see Phase 2).

- *medical or health concerns*: The therapist should get medical clearance for clients with a recent history of, or treatment for, stroke, heart attack, malignant hypertension, severe bronchial asthma, brain tumor, medical surgery, detached retina, delirium, or any other acute or serious, unstable medical condition (F. Shapiro, 2018).

- *seizure disorder*: Leeds (2009) reported that EMDR was safely used without the likelihood of initiating a genuine epileptic seizure. Pseudo-seizures from conversion or other medically unexplained conditions are fairly common in clients with a history of complex posttraumatic stress disorder (PTSD) or other severe traumatic stress injuries. Several EMDR case studies have been published on treating pseudoseizures (i.e., Kelley & Selim, 2007, as cited in Leeds, 2009).

- *traumatic brain injury (TBI)*: EMDR should not be used with clients presenting with acute (within days to a month) or severe TBI until they are medically cleared to engage in psychotherapy. For clients who have been medically cleared and/or present with a history of mild TBI (mTBI), EMDR therapy reprocessing should be considered. EMDR is a research-proven psychotherapeutic intervention that is effective in treating stress, anxiety, depression, and psychogenic pain. The emotional, behavioral, and physical impairments associated with mTBI can be successfully treated with EMDR (e.g., Jayatunge, 2013). In short,

EMDR may help address the past contributing traumatic events, current triggers related to the past trauma or recovery, and future-oriented client worry, concerns, or needed coping resources (Russell & Figley, 2013).

- *pregnancy*: All pregnant clients should be informed of the level of risk associated with increased stress from trauma-focused treatments. If there is a complicated pregnancy and/or the client is in the final trimester, it is recommended to postpone EMDR therapy reprocessing when possible (F. Shapiro, 2018).

- *severe psychopathology*: The common responses to clients with bipolar disorder, severe agitation or hostility, active suicidality, and psychoses is to stabilize and, where that is not possible, not use EMDR therapy. Start slowly and assess client reactions. Specific alternative protocols have been developed to guide EMDR therapists (Leeds, 2016; Parnell, 2006).

- *dissociative disorder*: Therapists should screen clients for dissociative identity disorder or other severe forms of dissociation. Special EMDR protocols have been developed for individuals with dissociative disorders (Knipe, 2015). In general, therapists are discouraged from using EMDR with this population unless under supervision with a provider experienced in the treatment of dissociation (F. Shapiro, 2018).

- *substance use disorder*: Clients with acute intoxication; with severe withdrawal symptoms such as delirium tremens, which is a medical emergency; or diagnosed with a severe life-threatening addiction are not suitable for EMDR therapy reprocessing. Specific EMDR protocols for addictive behaviors are available (Abel & O'Brien, 2014).

- *medication use*: Anecdotal reports of certain medications that may complicate reprocessing effects have arisen. The use of certain medications will prompt medical screening to determine the client's suitability for EMDR; these include lithium or Depakote (valproate) for bipolar disorder or digoxin for cardiac patients. The general rule of thumb for psychotropic medications is that reprocessing effects should be rechecked after the client tapers off the medication in the case of possible medication-induced distortion effects (F. Shapiro, 2018).

- *secondary gain*: Ordinarily, clients who are not truthful with the therapist will not benefit from treatment, including EMDR. There may be occasions when the client's blocking belief or motives for deception could be targeted for EMDR therapy reprocessing (Russell & Figley, 2013).

- *legal considerations*: Therapists entertaining EMDR therapy with crime victims, eyewitnesses, and first responders who may be required to testify or give legal disposition should be carefully informed of the potential risks and benefits of successful EMDR therapy and their pending legal involvement (F. Shapiro, 2018). Specifically, clients may have difficulty accessing a vivid picture or emotional response to the event of interest. Consider consultation with the client's attorney.

Readers are referred to F. Shapiro (2018) for further discussion about contraindications for EMDR therapy and actions the therapist might take to determine a client's readiness for EMDR therapy.

Treatment Planning

All psychotherapies use history taking to help determine the clinical picture before initiating therapy. Once a client is deemed suitable for EMDR therapy, the therapist identifies potential targets for reprocessing. Therapists must decide what client problems could be remediated via psychoeducation, problem solving, or teaching coping skills and what issues are more likely due to dysfunctionally stored information that could benefit from reprocessing. The therapist identifies the presenting complaint and its antecedents with as much specificity as possible, including the client's symptoms, duration of problems, initial onset (e.g., "When was the first time you can remember feeling this way?"), and additional past occurrences (e.g., "What other events have influenced the pathology?" "How could events be grouped together?" "Are themes emerging involving certain people, beliefs, and so forth?"; see F. Shapiro, 2018, for details).

Three-Pronged Protocol

While EMDR can treat many single-event trauma survivors by simply focusing on the targeted traumatic memory, many clients require a comprehensive treatment approach. The main goal of EMDR history taking and treatment planning is to identify the most salient past, current, and future experiential contributors of psychopathology, what we refer to as the *three-pronged protocol*:

- past traumatic events or other foundational emotionally charged experiential contributors, or small "t," that are etiologic to the presenting complaints or psychopathological condition;
- current internal or external triggers or antecedents that activate the maladaptive neural (memory) network; and
- future template of the client's anticipatory anxiety, worries, or concerns, and/or needed coping skills or mastery achieved through imaginal or behavioral rehearsal to prevent relapse, or reactivation, of the maladaptive schema (F. Shapiro, 2018).

Identifying Past Contributors

Presenting Complaint and Symptom History

At the outset of the clinical interview, clients are routinely asked to describe their current symptoms or complaints. Therapists should take careful notes of the language that clients use to describe their symptoms and problems and repeat that language back in future inquiries. The following is an example of using the client's presenting complaint to help identify possible past contributors for EMDR therapy reprocessing.

- *current onset*: "When did you first notice that you were not sleeping well, had no energy, and were being snappy?"

    Antecedents: "Do you know what might have caused this kind of reaction?" If not, "What was going on in your life when this started?"
- *earliest onset*: "When was the first time that you remember you felt this way?"

    Antecedents: "What was going on in your life back then when you had these same kinds of reactions?"
- *worst incident*: "Is this the worse it's ever been for you?"

    Antecedents: "What do you remember happening in your life that made this the worst time?"

These three sets of questions are used primarily to help select possible EMDR targets of past contributors to disturbance or psychopathology (Russell & Figley, 2013).

Earliest–Worst–Recent Reprocessing Sequence of Cluster Memories

According to the adaptive information processing (AIP) model, earlier traumas or adverse childhood experiences establish the foundation for reactions to subsequent life events. Therefore, with regard to treatment planning, the first target memory to reprocess is theoretically the earliest event, followed by the next earliest memory, and so on.

Memory Clusters. Clients are repeatedly exposed to a variety of potentially traumatic stressors. Experiences that are similar in some way—such as person, place, thing, event, emotion, physical sensation, behavioral response, and so on—become physiologically linked in the brain through the associative nature of memory networks. We call these *clusters* and posit that by targeting the earliest memory in the cluster, the worst incident in the cluster, and the most recent memory in the cluster, it is sufficient to process the remaining associated memories (F. Shapiro, 2018). Whether a combat veteran or a chronically abused child, therapy would be a lifelong proposition if every traumatic incident needed to be identified and reprocessed separately. Fortunately, it appears that EMDR produces a generalization effect that allows reprocessing to proceed more rapidly and efficiently by targeting the earliest, the "worst," and most recent memories. Clients who have difficulty identifying the worst memory of a cluster can be asked to identify one that best represents the others.

The earliest–worst–recent sequence makes sense intuitively because these are the events most likely to have the greatest emotional, somato-sensory, and cognitive impact. The main point is to identify a few, not all, of the most disturbing and therefore activating of memories in the maladaptive memory network. Anecdotally, EMDR therapists frequently report that other traumatic memories in the network have been reprocessed altogether or markedly reduced by focusing on the earliest–worst–recent sequence, but each therapist should check their work by instructing the client to check whether any other related memories are distressing and reprocess those accordingly (Russell & Figley, 2013).

Participant Cluster. Clusters of memories associated with a particular person (or particular persons)—such as the perpetrator of sexual molestation or abusive family members—who has etiological significance can be selected. Clients can be asked to picture the perpetrator's face and identify within the cluster of memories the earliest–worst–recent disturbing event (F. Shapiro, 2018).

Other EMDR-Related Considerations for Selecting Past Contributors

Starting With the "Worst" First. Therapists may want to start reprocessing the worst or most distressing presenting symptom first, instead of targeting the earliest, the conceptual preference. In most cases, the worst experience underlying the client's symptoms is usually what brought the client into treatment in the first place. By reprocessing memories associated with the most disturbing symptom, there is a better than even chance that symptom reduction or relief will be easily recognized by the client and possibly motivate the client to continue. A noticeable improvement in symptom relief and/or functioning is often vital to prevent premature termination. After the most debilitating symptom has been reprocessed, the therapist and client can then move on to the next most disturbing symptom, and so on.

I (M. C. R.) routinely start with the worst presenting symptom for the reasons stated earlier, and 80% to 90% of the time after the first reprocessing session, clients will report some measurable change in the narrative, image, cognition, feeling, and so forth—not a "cure" but a noticeably sufficient change that instills a sense of hope and a return appointment (e.g., F. Shapiro, 2018). I can think of no single case whereby a client treated with EMDR had reported some quota of change the first time and did not return for a subsequent appointment. Conversely, those few clients not reporting any alterations were notably less likely to keep their follow-up appointment (Russell & Figley, 2013).

Following the Client's Lead: Starting With the Least Versus Most Disturbing. Therapists often have a theory about the client's most salient memories of trauma and adverse experiences believed to be driving the current pathology. However, the therapist's view and the client's may not match. In this case, it is usually best to allow the client to take the lead as to what the client identifies as the most debilitating or meaningful target memory for initiating reprocessing. The therapist can place trust in the AIP model that neurophysiologically, whatever target memory is selected to begin processing will inevitably be associated with most of the other selected memories (Russell & Figley, 2013). Some clients express a preference to start EMDR therapy reprocessing gradually by choosing the least disturbing target memory and working their way up in a systematic desensitization format. This may be due to a fear of the unknown and whether they will be able to remain in control and not "lose it." Whatever the reason, therapists should respect the client's preference but also advise them that there is no guarantee that starting with the lesser upsetting events will not shift to the more disturbing experiences if the client is physically linked in a neural network. Clients who appear nervous about this proposition can be reminded of the information that will be covered in the preparation phase (Russell & Figley, 2013).

Feeder Memories. We use the term *feeder memories* to convey the idea that sometimes clients do not report and/or are not aware of earlier life experiences that may serve as "feeders" or contributors to the client's negative neural network. If identified, feeder memories should be incorporated into the treatment plan for reprocessing as early as possible (F. Shapiro, 2018).

Therapist Screening for a Feeder Memory

- *ask*: "When is the earliest time you remember feeling this way?" or "When is the earliest time you learned to think of yourself this way?"
- *float back*: "Bring up the picture and those words [negative cognition—NC]. Notice what feelings are coming up for you, where you are feeling them in your body, and just let your mind float back to an earlier time in your life. Don't search for anything, just let your mind float back, and tell me the earliest scene that comes to mind when you had similar thoughts, feelings, or sensations."

- *affect scan*: Use if the client cannot identify an NC. "Bring up the last time you felt upset. Hold the image in mind and the thoughts that come up about it. Where do you feel it in your body? Hold the image and the sensation, and let your mind scan back to the earliest time you remember feeling that way" (F. Shapiro, 2018).

Identifying Current Contributors

Triggers consist of any stimuli that elicit a response in the form of dysfunctional images, sensations, thoughts, or feelings associated with the earlier traumatic event(s). In soliciting the current triggers, therapists might ask, "Are there any things that you see, hear, think, or feel or certain situations or other reminders that seem to cause you to remember what happened or feel like it's happening again?" For treatment planning purposes, each trigger or antecedent needs to be reprocessed separately due to prior conditioning effects. For example, in a traumatic grief case from a motor vehicle accident where the client's wife died when a driver ran a light and slammed into the passenger side of their vehicle, the client's current triggers were (a) looking at family pictures; (b) the client's 13-year-old daughter, who has her mother's eyes; (c) anniversary dates (i.e., date of the accident, wedding anniversary, wife's birthday); (d) the sound of screaming; and (e) driving in traffic that invariably resulted in panic attack symptoms. Once all identified current precursors are reprocessed, the therapist moves on to reprocessing the anticipatory anxieties or other future-oriented stimuli related to future client coping and self-efficacy. There are several procedures used to help identify appropriate target memories for EMDR processing. After all the current triggers have been reprocessed, the therapist then proceeds to the future template.

Identifying Future Contributors

The therapist identifies future behaviors necessary for appropriate future action, including strengthening associations of the client's desired state in terms of how the client would like to be thinking, feeling, or acting in the future, as well as reducing anticipatory anxiety, worrying, or self-handicapping behaviors related to future performance (Russell & Figley, 2013; F. Shapiro, 2018). Clients are asked, "How do you see yourself coping with this problem in the future?" "What would you like to be doing, thinking, or feeling, or how would you like to be reacting in the future?" "What new skills or ways of thinking about things will you need?" One or two items are typically identified, but however many, each is reprocessed separately. The reprocessing phase is concluded after the last future contributor has been reprocessed and checked. With regard to the afore-mentioned motor vehicle case study, the client's future template consisted of (a) being able to relish the positive memories of his wife, (b) being able to feel and express a father's love for his daughter, and (c) feeling comfortable driving a car without extreme anxiety.

Using the AIP model as our guide, by identifying several of the most hotly charged memories in the maladaptive neural network, the therapist can reasonably expect generalization effects to other associatively linked memories. Therefore, in EMDR, we do not need nor want to identify and reprocess every incident. The treatment plan that the therapist may typically start with is often not the treatment plan at the end. New or previously undisclosed recollections (or "progressions") regularly emerge during EMDR and may become targets (Russell & Figley, 2013).

Traumatic Stress Injury and Comorbidity

Comorbid medical, medically unexplained, and neuropsychiatric conditions are important to recognize and differentiate because they can modify clinical determinations of prognosis, treatment priorities, selection of interventions, and the setting where care may be provided. For example, according to the Department of Veterans Affairs (DVA) and Department of Defense (2017) PTSD guidelines, therapists should anticipate that at least 50% to 80% of veterans with traumatic stress injuries (i.e., PTSD) will have one or more coexisting mental health disorder, such as dementia, depression, substance abuse or withdrawal, insomnia, bereavement, psychosis, seizure disorder, TBI, thyroid disease, neoplasm, and/or medically unexplained conditions (i.e., headaches, irritable bowel, chronic fatigue, noncardiac chest pain). The same level of comorbidity can be expected in clients exposed to traumatic stressors other than war. Clients presenting with co-occurring disorders, such as depression and alcohol abuse, are at much greater risk of suicide and interpersonal violence than clients with only one war stress injury. The following are general recommendations for screening clients for comorbidities:

- Pain (acute and chronic) and sleep disturbances should be assessed in all patients with PTSD.
- Generalized physical and cognitive health symptoms—also attributed to concussion or mTBI and many other causes—should be assessed and managed in patients with PTSD and a co-occurring diagnosis of mTBI.
- Associated high-risk behaviors (e.g., smoking, alcohol or drug abuse, unsafe weapon storage, dangerous driving, HIV, and hepatitis risks) should be assessed in patients with PTSD. Providers should consider the existence of comorbid conditions when deciding whether to treat patients in the primary care setting or refer them for specialty mental health care.
- Clients with complicated comorbidities may be referred to mental health or PTSD specialty care for evaluation and diagnosis (Russell & Figley, 2013).

Research has shown that EMDR therapy is often effective in simultaneously treating a wide range of co-occurring conditions, including but not limited to depressive disorders, anxiety disorders, medically unexplained physical symptoms, pain-related conditions, traumatic grief, moral injury, posttraumatic anger, dissociation, phantom-limb pain and sensations, and so forth (e.g., Russell & Figley, 2013; F. Shapiro, 2018).

PHASE 2: CLIENT PREPARATION

After completing Phase 1, deeming a client as suitable and developing a treatment plan, the therapist next prepares the client for reprocessing. The preparation stage establishes the therapeutic framework and client expectations so that clients can safely manage their level of distress that predictably will emerge during reprocessing. The therapist readies the client for EMDR therapy by strengthening the collaborative therapeutic alliance, identifying common goals, and soliciting honest communication between the client and therapist.

Adopting a Clinical Stance and Establishing the Therapeutic Alliance

To facilitate the healing process, the therapist needs to communicate to the client a sense of respect for and importance of the client's safety. Establishing a trusting and effective therapeutic alliance is crucial in psychotherapy in general but especially in trauma-focused treatments such as EMDR, the absence of which is contraindicated for any trauma work. In preparing the client for reprocessing, the therapist strives to instill a sense of collaboration. The duration of the preparation phase will vary from client to client. In some cases, an effective alliance can be established within one to two sessions; others, especially with complex trauma or those predisposed to be more mistrusting of others, may take longer to form that bond. Therapists should monitor whether the client's self-reports might suggest an attempt to please the therapist or prematurely end treatment. In doing so, it is essential that clients are advised to provide honest self-reports whether they are experiencing changes or not.

Therapists need to ensure that the client appreciates the importance of accurate self-reporting during and between sessions by giving instructions such as the following: "All you need to do is tell me the truth about what you are experiencing so I can make the proper choices. Just give me accurate feedback about what is happening. Also, you are the one in control. If you need to stop, just let me know. Just tell me what is happening for you."

Explaining the Adaptive Information Processing Model

Therapists need to offer the client a general explanation of trauma, the AIP model, and EMDR therapy procedures using language clients can understand (e.g., Gomez, 2013; Russell & Figley, 2013; F. Shapiro, 2018). It is usually best to provide brief descriptions such as, "When a trauma occurs, it appears to get locked in the brain" and that "this information becomes easily triggered by various reminders" and is why the client feels the way they do (e.g., a sense of hopelessness, headaches, tension, anxiety). Similarly, clients can be told that eye movements in EMDR appear to mimic what occurs in rapid eye movement (REM) sleep; however, doing the eye movements while awake and conscious versus asleep allows for greater reprocessing of negative information. Preparing clients for EMDR can include a description of the AIP model such as the following:

> Often, when something traumatic happens, it seems to get locked in the nervous system with the original picture, sounds, thoughts, feelings, and so on. Because the experience is locked there, it continues to be triggered whenever a reminder comes up. It can be the basis for a lot of discomfort and sometimes a lot of negative emotions, such as fear and helplessness, that we can't seem to control. These are really the emotions connected with the old experience that are being triggered. The eye movements we use in EMDR seem to unlock the nervous system and allow your brain to process the experience. That may be what is happening in REM, or dream, sleep: The eye movements may be involved in processing the unconscious material. The important thing to remember is that your brain will be doing the healing, and you are the one in control. (F. Shapiro, 2018)

Demonstrating the Mechanics of Eye Movement Desensitization and Reprocessing

After arranging the chairs in the classic "ships passing in the night" arrangement (whereby the therapist, if they are right-handed, will place their chair facing the client but off to the left side from the therapist's perspective, and vice versa for left-handed therapists), the therapist also introduces BLS to clients. For eye movements, the therapist collaborates with the client to determine the comfortable distance and direction of eye movement by asking, "Where does it feel most comfortable to have my hand?" The distance from the visual stimulus to the client should not be so far (more than four feet) that the client's visual field is occupied by background distractions.

Bilateral Stimulation Using Visual Stimulus and Eye Movements

Using the therapist's hand or a wand, start with the therapist's hand in the center of the face; slowly move laterally, side-by-side, reminding the client to track only with their eyes; and speed up the hand movements until the client is unable to track them. The therapist can test out diagonal movements (left to upper right). Vertical eye movement is anecdotally reported as helpful for dizziness or vertigo.

Several electronic device options exist that produce BLS (e.g., light bars with lights that are tracked from left to right). When using an electronic device, therapists should start with a slow speed and increase to find the upper limit of client tracking. Most clients prefer and respond best to a faster BLS rate. No studies have been conducted comparing the relative potential benefits, drawbacks, or effectiveness of BLS delivered manually (i.e., hand waving) or by electronic device.

Bilateral Stimulation Using Auditory Sounds

- Alternate opening and closing the hand.
- When using electronic devices and headphones, offer alternating sounds. Adolescents and young adults often seem to prefer using headphones. No research exists comparing the relative benefits or drawbacks of generating auditory stimuli manually or via electronic device.

Bilateral Stimulation Using Kinesthetic Vibrations or Taps

- Alternating finger taps were used with a control group for testing the effects of eye movements in one of the first DVA random clinical trials on EMDR.
- *alternating tapping*: On a trip to Central America, therapist Priscilla Marquis was working with blind survivors of land mines. Eye movements were not feasible, so the therapist had clients hold out their

hands, and the therapist tapped alternately either the hand or knee, which demonstrated that BLS other than eye movements could be used successfully.

- *"butterfly hug"*: Researchers with young children after natural disasters reported that this technique was effective. The child is asked to wrap their arms around themselves and alternate taps on their backsides or shoulders under clinical supervision (e.g., Fernandez, 2007).
- *electronic devices and alternating vibration pads*: Clients hold onto pads in their hands that generate alternating vibrating sensations. No research exists comparing the relative benefits or drawbacks of generating auditory stimuli manually or via electronic device.

Combining Stimuli

I (M. C. R.) provided anecdotal case studies combining BLS (visual, auditory, and/or kinesthetic) with positive effects when clients did not respond to eye movements or other stimuli alone (Russell & Figley, 2013). However, the combination of BLS has yet to be researched.

Affect Tolerance and Instilling a Safe and Calm Place

As mentioned in Phase 1, therapists are recommended to use relaxation techniques such as the safe and calm place exercise for prospective EMDR clients to determine a client's capacity for self-regulation, which will be important immediately after and between EMDR therapy reprocessing sessions. A description of the eight-step safe and calm place exercise can be found in Appendix B.

Clarifying Client and Therapist Role Expectations

The standard EMDR description of the client's expectations goes something like this:

> What we will be doing is a simple check on what you are experiencing. I need to know from you what is going on with as clear feedback as possible. Sometimes things will change, and sometimes they won't.

I'll ask you how you feel from 0 to 10—sometimes it will change, and sometimes it won't. I may ask if something else comes up—sometimes it will, and sometimes it won't. There are no "supposed to's" in this process. So just give as accurate feedback as you can as to what's happening without judging whether it should be happening or not. Just let whatever happens happen. We'll do the eye movement for a while, and then we'll talk about it. (F. Shapiro, 2018)

Another way of explaining the client's role is the following:

All I need is for you to tell me the truth about what you are experiencing. I don't need to know all the details—that's up to you to decide how much to tell me—but at a minimum, we need your honest feedback if things are changing or not. Please don't try to force yourself to concentrate on a certain memory, picture, or whatever; just be an observer and notice whatever it is that comes. Just notice it. Remember, you've got the controls, so if you want me to stop, you're the boss. (Russell & Figley, 2013)

Introducing Metaphor for Expected Client Roles During Reprocessing

EMDR therapists often use a train metaphor to describe "mindful noticing," whereby clients are instructed to recall looking out of a train window and watching the scenery. For many of us, this is a powerful metaphor. Increasingly, however, younger generations, at least in the United States, do not have the experience of riding in a train. They could imagine what it would be like, but it would not likely be as strong an experience as for those who had been on a train. Consequently, with younger cohorts, using the metaphor of looking out of the window of a car will unquestionably be an experience to which they can relate.

To designate a *stop signal*, clients are asked to identify a nonverbal way to communicate their desire that the therapist ends the BLS set. Clients are instructed, "If you need to stop, raise your hand, and I will immediately stop, and we will discuss what is happening and decide what we do from there." It is essential that clients understand that they are in charge and have control, and they have not failed if they need to stop.

Most adolescents and adults have had the experience of driving a vehicle; hence, the *brake and gas pedal metaphor* can be useful for instilling a sense of control and safety during reprocessing. Once the client's stop signal is established, the brake and gas pedal metaphor are introduced. In short, clients are advised that when the therapist starts using BLS, the clients are in the driver's seat. The brake is their stop signal, and BLS is the gas pedal. Clients are advised that keeping their foot on the gas pedal will get them to their destination quicker, and conversely, using the brake will slow their arrival. Nevertheless, all cars have a brake and gas pedal for a reason, so clients can use them as they see fit. Therapists who use this metaphor will find it useful for clients who frequently want to verbally process their experiences, sometimes for lengthy periods. There are many conceivable reasons clients would choose to do so, and the therapist should respect their desire. However, when stopping and talking and more talking becomes the norm, one way to reset the norm is to remind them of the gas pedal. If the pattern continues, therapists will need to assess for a possible blocking belief (Russell & Figley, 2013).

Resource Development and Installation

Client history taking may reveal that certain clients are too unstable or not currently ready for reprocessing due to temporary time constraints, emotional or behavioral instability, or poor self-regulation skills. Resource development and installation (RDI) was developed by Debra Korn and Andrew Leeds (2002) as a means to enhance or strengthen the client's access to internal "resources" or sources of resilience associated with their adaptive neural networks. RDI uses the client's positive emotions and life experiences needed to cope with challenging situations, including trauma-focused reprocessing. These resources include positive emotions (e.g., confidence, competency, mastery, enjoyment) and adaptive reactions of others whom the client admires or strongly identifies with (e.g., actors, athletes, relatives, close friends), as well as the client's own examples of successful adaptation (e.g., sporting achievements, getting a good grade in a difficult class). It is critical that therapists do not confuse RDI with EMDR. The former is intended to help prepare clients for trauma-focused work (Korn & Leeds, 2002). Additional examples of possible client resources include the following:

- *mastery*: experience of past coping, self-care, or a self-soothing stance or movement that evokes a needed state
- *relationship*: positive role models
  - memories of supportive others
- *symbolic*: natural objects that represent the needed attribute
  - symbols from dreams, daydreams, or guided imagery
  - cultural, religious, or spiritual symbols
  - metaphors
  - music
  - images of a positive goal state or future self

Length and Pace of Eye Movement Desensitization and Reprocessing Treatment Sessions

It has been recommended that EMDR sessions last 90 minutes from the beginning; this length is still taught as the preferred meeting duration to ensure sufficient time to complete reprocessing. However, in many health care settings, particularly managed care and the military, providers often do not have the liberty, nor might it be feasible if they did, to use the extended session format. Fortunately, a large, well-controlled study on EMDR in a managed-care setting has been conducted. Marcus et al. (1997) compared 67 adult clients diagnosed with PTSD who received either 50-minute individual EMDR; psychodynamic, cognitive, or behavior therapy; or group therapy at a Kaiser Permanente hospital. The results demonstrated not only that EMDR can be implemented effectively within a standard 50-minute therapy format but also that clients receiving EMDR reported significantly lower symptoms of PTSD, depression, and anxiety than clients from the other treatment groups, with an average of 6.5 sessions versus 11.8 sessions. Moreover, 77% of EMDR clients no longer met diagnostic criteria, with most treatment gains maintained at 6-month follow-up (Markus et al., 2004; Russell & Figley, 2013).

PHASE 3: ASSESSMENT

The key to psychological change is the ability to facilitate appropriate information processing (F. Shapiro, 2018). In collaboration with the client during Phase 1, a number of past events, current triggers, and future-oriented goals that are believed to be the principal cause of the client's presenting complaint and suffering have been identified. According to the AIP model, traumatic or highly upsetting memories often include an image or other sensory elements (e.g., sound, taste, smells), emotions, physical reactions, and cognitions at the time of the event that link to similar experiences in one's neural memory network. In EMDR, assessment is not concerned with diagnosis per se but with identifying relevant information for each memory that will be targeted and activated during reprocessing. However, before actual reprocessing can commence, the therapist must complete two vital tasks:

- identify the critical core components of each target memory and
- obtain baseline measures for each target memory.

Successful EMDR treatment does not require the client to disclose all the specifics of the target memory, and the therapist should not pressure clients to reveal more than they are comfortable with (F. Shapiro, 2018). Moreover, not all clients will be able to identify an example of each memory component. Nevertheless, EMDR therapy reprocessing can proceed. After the client has identified the memory to be targeted, the therapist inquires, "What happens when you think of the incident?" or "When you think of the incident, what do you get?" The client's answer provides the therapist with some insight into how their brain is presently storing the traumatic information; by Phase 8, the identical questions should solicit a notably different reaction.

Case Example

The client is a 38-year-old adult who was sexually groomed and assaulted when they were 16 years old by a high school basketball coach. In addition to suffering symptoms of PTSD and depression, the client reports significant difficulty trusting others and themselves by harboring self-blame for the event. We use this case to illustrate the various assessment steps. That said, the following assessment procedures are designed to gather sufficient information required for EMDR therapy reprocessing.

Selecting the Image

The first component to be identified is the sensory memory of the event. For most people, this will be a visual image or picture: "What picture best represents the experience or incident to you?" Clients will often report a litany of images associated with the disturbing memory (e.g., the sight of an oncoming vehicle, image of a combat buddy's mutilated body, picture of a perpetrator's face); indeed, most of our declarative memories have a beginning, middle, and end. So, the therapist might ask, "What picture represents the worst part of the experience as you think about it now?" (see Exhibit 4.1).

If the client is unable to identify a particular image, possibly due to dissociation, the therapist should ask the client to "think of the incident." Simply "thinking of the event" often leads to the client accessing and stimulating the targeted information.

Exhibit 4.1

Soliciting the Image

Therapist: What picture represents the worst part of the experience as you think about it now?

Client: I see my coach's face. He is smirking at me after he raped me, like I mean nothing to him.

Moreover, when clients are unable to identify a specific image of the incident or a representative image of a cluster of incidents, there is an excellent chance that the most prominent sensory memory is not an image but maybe a smell, sound, pain, or taste. For example, I (M. C. R.) treated a survivor of a motor vehicle accident who sustained a traumatic brain injury and suffered anterograde amnesia. The client could not recall the memory of the event, so there was no image of the memory accessible. What the client did recall was a "sickly sweet smell" that they continued to smell in the hospital and after they returned home. The odor was blood. If clients cannot identify an image, the therapist might ask, "When you think of the experience, what do you notice now?" If they struggle, the therapist can prompt, "Is there a particular sound, smell, or taste that stands out?"

The following are other sensory memories that people may experience (Russell & Figley, 2013):

- Audition (sounds)
    - explosions
    - gunfire, ricochets, and near misses
    - cries of wounded people
    - sirens
    - crushing metal
    - whistling of incoming rounds
    - pleas for help or mercy
    - wailing of mourners
    - shouts of rage and taunts
    - multiple commands
- Olfaction (smells)
    - rotting garbage
    - burnt flesh and hair
    - heavy chemical and industrial smoke or fuel
    - alcohol
    - open sewage, feces, and stale urine
    - decaying animals

- gun powder
- burning rubber
- Gustatory (tastes)
  - metallic (adrenaline)
  - fishy (semen)

Identifying the Negative Cognition

After identifying the sensory memory of the target, the therapist now solicits the client's negative, self-denigrating self-statement linked to the incident. Memories of disturbing events from the distant past, when stimulated, often cause dysfunction and distress that contribute to the client's negative self-appraisals. Clients are instructed to bring up the memory and the image or another sensory memory they reported and are asked: "What words go best with the picture that express your negative belief about yourself now?" Or the therapist can ask, "When you think of that picture, what do you believe about yourself now?" "What does that say about you as a person?" (see Exhibit 4.2).

Ideally, the NC will be a negative, self-referencing, irrational, and presently held belief that accurately focuses the client's presenting issue, generalizes to related events or concerns, and resonates with the client's

---

Exhibit 4.2

Soliciting the Negative Cognition

Therapist: What belief about yourself goes with that picture?

Client: I should have never trusted him. [Perhaps this is a valid statement of fact, but it does not reflect a currently held negative self-belief.]

Therapist: Okay, but when you think of that image of your coach smirking at you, what do you believe about yourself now?

Client: I'm dirty!

---

affect. During EMDR training, participants are taught to aim for an "I" statement—ergo the "self-referencing" feature—and the negative belief should be related to what they believe about themselves in the present—"now"—as they recollect what happened. What are therapists to do should clients report five NCs? The therapist can ask, "Which one stands out for you and really represents your belief about yourself now?" In other words, the EMDR therapist wants one, and only one, NC. Trainees are also advised about what makes a poor choice for an NC, such as a description of the past ("It was awful"), a feeling statement ("I'm pissed"), or wishful thinking ("He shouldn't have died"). What is the EMDR therapist really after?

The purpose of the NC is to identify the most prominent, affect-laden cognition in the maladaptive neural network. By its nature, the self-referencing "I am worthless, a coward, weak [and so forth]" statement is more likely to generalize to other beliefs about the self and other adverse events. Such a core belief will be associated with affect. The stronger the belief, the stronger the affect, and this allows the client greater "access" to the existing maladaptive neural network and is more likely to be linked to other similar networks during reprocessing. That is the ideal NC. Therapists familiar with cognitive therapy may have fewer problems with "peeling the onion" to get to the negative core belief.

Now we will contradict ourselves. The search for the perfect NC—self-referencing, present focused, and generalizable—is theoretically optimal, but it may not be the most relevant to the client. It has been observed on frequent occasions when therapists get wrapped up in soliciting the ideal "I" statement, frustrating their client and themselves and delaying or derailing treatment. Remember, the ultimate goal is to identify a single representative, powerful NC that is affect laden and prominent in the etiology of the client's condition and therefore will help the client access the maladaptive neural network. Access to the maladaptive network generally means the therapist and client have access to other memories, sensory images, cognitions, emotions, and sensations because they are physiologically linked. That means the cognitions from the onion peeled earlier were most assuredly in the same neural net.

Clients who have difficulty identifying an NC on their own can be asked to select a potential NC from a list, as presented in Appendix D.

Selecting a Positive Cognition

After obtaining the NC, the therapist solicits a self-referencing belief that addresses the same concern as the NC, accurately focuses the client's desired direction of change, is initially acceptable, and can generalize to related events or concerns. Ideally, the positive cognition (PC) is diametrically opposite of the NC. For example, an NC of "I am weak" might lead to a PC of "I am strong." The therapist solicits the PC by saying, "When you bring up that picture (or experience) what would you prefer to believe about yourself now instead?" Like the NC, the PC is not an absolute or magical unrealistic thought about changing events or attributes ("I will never fail again") and should be worded positively to avoid confusion: "I am strong" rather than "I am not weak" (see Exhibit 4.3).

Soliciting the PC provides us a window into the realm of adaptive possibilities. If a client enters our office and the therapist works with them to resolve their particular problem, irrespective of EMDR, what would be the adaptive resolution we hope clients reach? For a client with PTSD from a motor vehicle accident 5 years ago when no serious injuries were sustained by either party, it might be something such as, "It's over now; it's in the past. I survived; life goes on." In EMDR, the therapist has the client look into their crystal ball and ask what their adaptive resolution would be for their situation. There are several reasons the therapist might want to do this. One is to determine whether the client can access more adaptive neural networks that store mastery, secure attachment, past success, coping resources, and the like. Accessing the adaptive memory network is what EMDR therapy reprocessing is all about. When the client's maladaptive neural networks are activated—for example, in PTSD—it dominates the client's attentional focus, cognitive capacity, emotional regulation, sleep, and so on. The adaptive neural networks cannot compete because the brain–body is in full survivor mode. The EMDR therapist invites the client to access the adaptive neural networks, and by doing so,

---

Exhibit 4.3

Soliciting the Positive Cognition

Therapist: When you bring up that picture of your coach smirking at you, what would you prefer to believe about yourself now instead?

Client: I don't know . . . that it wasn't my fault, that I'm not dirty!

Therapist: Which of those two statements "it wasn't my fault" and "I'm not dirty" is the strongest one you would like to believe about yourself now?

Client: I'm not dirty.

Therapist: And what would that mean if you're not dirty? [In an attempt to avoid a negative in the PC.]

Client: That I'm a good person.

Therapist: How does "I'm a good person" sound?

Client: Yes, sounds good.

---

we are now linking the two neural networks. The second reason therapists solicit the PC is that it provides a measure of how demoralized the client is. If they can entertain for a few minutes an adaptive response to their inner turmoil, there is reason to hope. When clients are unable to come up with any PC, a therapist should assess for dangerousness and probably consider RDI for the time being. Why assess for dangerousness? The single strongest predictor for suicide is the absence of hope (Russell & Figley, 2013).

As with the NC, if clients are unable to identify an appropriate PC on their own, the therapist can ask them to select a PC from a table such as the one in Appendix D. Therapists should bear in mind that whatever PC the client may start with, it is subject to change once reprocessing commences. It is quite common after successful EMDR therapy that the client's new, subsequent PC is more adaptive than the original PC selected before treatment ensues. For instance, I (M. C. R.) had a 22-year-old male client, "Jim," who had PTSD and phantom limb pain (PLP) following a traumatic leg amputation (Russell, 2008b). Jim adamantly insisted that his initial PC was "I'm alive," so I went with that. By the sixth and final EMDR session that led to a significant boost in self-esteem and decrease in his PTSD and PLP symptoms, Jim was asked to recall the original target memory and whether the words "I'm alive" still fit. He immediately shot back, "No, I want to change that to 'I'm strong.'" In other words, Jim's PC shifted from a description of surviving the trauma to an infinitely more adaptive and generalizable core belief, "I'm strong." Many, if not most, EMDR therapists will have similar clinical outcomes.

Rating the Validity of Cognition

Now, the therapist comes to one of the two baseline measures for the target memories. The validity of cognition (VOC) is intended to be a measure of the client's felt confidence in their adaptive self-statement. How strongly do they feel in their gut that "I am a protector?" So, the therapist asks, "When you think of the memory, how true do those words [*repeat the PC*] feel to you now on a scale from 1 to 7, where 1 feels completely false and 7 feels completely true?" Occasionally, it may be helpful to explain to clients, "Remember, sometimes we know something with our head, but it feels differently in our gut. In this case, what is the gut-level feeling of the truth of [*repeat the PC*], from 1 (*completely false*) to 7 (*completely true*)?" (see Exhibit 4.4).

If the initial VOC is a 1, the therapist should consider the appropriateness of the PC and check for an alternative PC. If the client offers multiple ratings ("I think it's maybe a 1½ or 2"), the therapist needs to keep things simple by saying, "If you had to pick one or the other, which feels truer about yourself now, 1½ or 2?" The VOC provides a useful baseline for the sense of hopefulness and adaptive possibilities on the horizon. More precisely, the simple 1–7 VOC rating gives the therapist and client an estimation of the relative strength of the tentative association between the maladaptive and adaptive neural networks. Therapists should be aware

---

Exhibit 4.4

Obtaining the VOC

Therapist: When you think of the memory, how true do those words "I'm a good person" feel to you now on a scale from 1 to 7, where 1 feels completely false, and 7 feels completely true?

Client: Maybe a 3. I know I'm a good person, but when I think about what happened, it still bothers me that I let it happen.

Therapist: So, a 3?

Client: Yes.

---

that throughout the assessment phase, clients are progressively accessing their traumatic or distressing memories, which is why the therapist prepares the client during Phase 2.

Identifying Emotions

After accessing the adaptive neural networks by soliciting and measuring the PC, the therapist redirects the client's self-focus to the maladaptive neural network and, specifically, the target memory by asking, "When you think of the memory and the words [*repeat the NC*], what emotions do you feel now?" Again, as with the NC and PC, the EMDR therapist is interested in how the information is presently stored in memory, not what emotions existed at the time of the incident. Accessing the client's image, NC, and emotions associated with the target memory permits us to efficiently obtain the second baseline measure of the client's level of distress. Clients are requested to identify specific emotions linked to the target memory, and the therapist records those emotions without further questioning or narrowing them down to a single emotion. Numbness and emptiness are emotional states and should be recorded as such (Russell & Figley, 2013; see Exhibit 4.5).

Exhibit 4.5

Soliciting Emotions

Therapist: When you think of the memory and the words "I'm dirty," what emotions do you feel now?

Client: I feel sad . . . angry . . . embarrassed . . . and probably ashamed.

Therapist: Okay. [The therapist records all emotions the client identifies.]

Estimating the Subjective Units of Disturbance

Immediately after the client names their emotions, the therapist follows with "On a scale of 0 to 10, where 0 is no disturbance or neutral and 10 is the highest disturbance you can imagine, how disturbing does it feel now?" If the client identifies several emotions, the subjective units of disturbance (SUD) rating is based only on the total distress, not each emotion. The SUD baseline serves to alert both the therapist and client about the current level of disturbance. If the client offers multiple SUD ratings ("About an 8 or 9" or "between 8 to 10"), the therapist should ask, "If you have to pick one, which SUD rating best describes how distressed you feel about the memory right now?" (see Exhibit 4.6).

Exhibit 4.6

Obtaining the SUD Scale

Therapist: On a scale of 0 to 10, where 0 is no disturbance or neutral and 10 is the highest disturbance you can imagine, how disturbing does it feel now?

Client: Now? Maybe a 2.

The therapist should be prepared for client ratings that may not always match the content of their narrative—for example, sometimes clients will report an SUD rating that appears to be incongruent. For instance, a witness to a terrorist bombing reported images of "body parts and blood everywhere" but gave an SUD rating of "about a 2 or 3." The lower-than-expected subjective rating may be a sign of the client's previous level of exposure or habituation to such scenes (e.g., first responder), or the client may be restricting their attentional focus to control the amount of exposure to the scene for self-protective reasons, or they may be experiencing a numb, dissociative state, among other plausible explanations. At this point, the therapist should not challenge the client's self-ratings as long as they are above a 2, meaning that they are two clicks above zero and reflect some measure of disturbance. Therapists can anticipate that a low SUD rating at assessment does not predict the level of disturbance during reprocessing because it will invariably increase.

Identifying Body (Somatic) Sensations

Again, without delay, immediately after obtaining the SUD rating, the therapist says, "Where do you feel it [the disturbance] in your body?" Somatic or physical sensations are a common response to trauma and thus play a critical role in trauma-focused therapies such as EMDR. Even when clients identify emotions such as "emptiness," "pain," or "numbness," the therapist should ask, "And where in your body do you feel [the emotion] the most?" Clients may report a location or diffuse sensation throughout their body. No matter what is said, the therapist records it. Like emotions, clients can report as many physical sensations as they see fit. The therapist does not need to do or say anything other than record what the clients say and the location (see Exhibit 4.7).

When clients report multiple physical symptoms, it is not necessary for the therapist to map out each one. The therapist can repeat back all the physical sensations the client reported and simply ask, "Where do you feel these in your body?" Clients may describe each sensation and its location, but most times they may report locations but not specify which sensation is where. In the grand scheme of the EMDR assessment, locating each

---

Exhibit 4.7

Obtaining Body Sensations

Therapist: And where do you feel it [the disturbance] in your body? [This is done right after soliciting the SUD rating.]

Client: [*Places their hand on their abdomen*] In my stomach area. Also, my neck is tight, and I have a little headache.

---

specific physical sensation is not necessary, nor is it helpful for the therapist to ask for elaboration about the sensations reported. A client who has difficulty identifying the location of the somatic symptoms may need some assistance from the therapist by referring to their SUD rating and saying, "You reported an 8 on the SUD scale. Where do you feel the 9 in your body?" If the client still struggles with this, the therapist can acknowledge that many clients have troubles with this kind of question and instruct them as follows:

> Close your eyes and notice how your body feels. Now I will ask you to think of something, and when I do, just notice what changes in your body. Okay, notice your body. Now, think of (or bring up the picture of) the memory. Tell me what changes. Now add the words [*repeat the NC*]. Tell me what changes.

Most clients will be able to report some muscle tightening or tension or increased heart or breathing rate. No matter how small, the client's physical sensations should be documented and targeted. There are times where the client's physical sensations are the primary and sometimes near-exclusive focus during reprocessing (e.g., Russell, 2008b).

PHASE 4: DESENSITIZATION

In Phase 4 (as well as 5 & 6), the therapist and client implement the EMDR therapy reprocessing treatment plan by incorporating eye movements or alternative forms of BLS. We recommend that the therapist use eye movements for BLS whenever possible (F. Shapiro, 2018). In short, there have been over 30 trials documenting significant therapeutic benefits with eye movements in decreasing arousal and memory vividness and/or negative affect (e.g., Barrowcliff et al., 2004; Lee & Cuijpers, 2013), increasing recognition of factual information (Parker et al., 2009), retrieving episodic memories (Christman et al., 2003), and achieving attentional flexibility (Kuiken et al., 2001). The goal of the desensitization phase is to reduce the client's level of disturbance (when possible) to an SUD rating of 0 or 1, if ecologically valid (e.g., death of a loved one). The term *desensitization* is misleading in that it describes a reprocessing byproduct. It is necessary to process dysfunctional information linked to the target memory (or memories), and this is accomplished by the BLS (e.g., eye movements).

Accelerated Reprocessing of Memories

Immediately after identifying the location of body sensations in the EMDR assessment phase, the therapist informs the client about the nature of EMDR processing and the fact that seemingly unrelated memories can be stimulated during reprocessing. Importantly, clients are reminded to just notice and report whatever comes up:

> Now remember, it is your brain that is doing the healing, and you are the one in control. I will ask you to mentally focus on the target and follow my finger with your eyes. Just let whatever happens happen, and we will talk at the end of the set. Just tell me what comes up, and don't discard anything as unimportant. Any new information that comes to mind is connected in some way. If you want to stop, just raise your hand [or whatever stop signal was decided in Phase 2].

After the reminder, the therapist instructs the client to bring up the image and NC and notice the body sensations as reported in Phase 3: "Bring up the picture and the words [*repeat the NC*] and notice where you feel it in your body. Now, follow my fingers with your eyes."

Focusing on all three memory components at the same time is intended to form an initial link to the dysfunctional memory. The therapist then initiates a set of 24 rapid, left-to-right eye movements or alternating BLS (hereafter, we use the term BLS) in a horizontal manner. Once the BLS is started, new sensory elements, beliefs, emotions, and somatic sensations will inevitably emerge. Clients should be told not to try to hold onto the image of the target memory during the BLS because new information is bound to be stimulated (F. Shapiro, 2018). The speed of the BLS is whatever the client can handle. If using eye movements, the therapist may observe the client having constant trouble tracking the therapist's hand (or light device is used) and/or complaining about the speed of the external stimulus or feeling "dizzy" or other uncomfortable physical sensation that they relate to the speed of the BLS. When this occurs, the therapist should try a slower speed.

However, it is critical that the therapist reminds the client not to force themselves to focus on any one memory or component (e.g., image) because this can stall reprocessing; the therapist should repeat, "Just let whatever happens, happen; just notice it." Therapists who forget to remind the client during the initial BLS sets may see the client struggle to track the speed of the BLS due to their efforts to forcibly hold onto the original image of the target memory versus "just letting what happens, happen."

During the BLS, therapists should softly give the client external feedback by periodically saying "Good," "That's it," "Just notice it." Per the AIP model, the EMDR therapist believes the therapist's verbalizations serve to enhance the dual-focused component instead of engaging in excessive self-focus or absorption in the traumatic material, which can be overwhelming for some clients. The therapist's verbal refrains also serve the purpose of conveying a sense of safety and reassurance to the client.

At the end of the BLS set, clients are instructed to "Let it go or blank it out, and take a deep breath." To avoid a possible immersion into dissociation or a trance-like state, the therapist should not direct the client to close their eyes as they take a breath. The refocusing intervals between BLS sets allow clients to briefly interrupt the intensity of reprocessing by giving the client permission to reorient, rest, and prepare to report to the therapist about the experiential changes that occurred during reprocessing. These brief interludes also permit clients to gain a sense of control over their inner experience with the traumatic or distressing material. Therapists also may find themselves unintentionally or intentionally pacing their own breathing with the client's; this is encouraged in the context of self-care.

After the client (and therapist) takes a breath, the therapist reestablishes contact by saying, "What do you get now?" or "What are you noticing now?" The open-ended questioning allows clients to share whatever information they want with the therapist. If the client struggles to answer the initial prompting, the therapist can ask, "What came up for you?" The purpose of this open line of questioning is to solicit feedback from the client about any changes in images, thoughts, sensations, or feelings within the target memory or a shifting to other associated memories. Therapists using closed-ended questions such as "What has changed?" may create a demand characteristic implying to the client that failure to report change connotes something amiss. Therapists should also avoid questions such as "What do you see now?" or "What are you feeling?" at the end of a BLS set, in that per the AIP model, the most salient change could be a belief, an insight, or body sensation. If the client replies "Nothing," the therapist instructs the client to think about the target memory again: "When you think of the incident, what do you get?"

Due to the highly individualized effects of reprocessing, the EMDR therapist asks, "What do you get now?" allowing the client to report any dominant shifts in images, emotions, cognition, or somatic sensations or a change to another memory altogether. If the client's self-report indicates a change, the therapist instructs the client to "Focus on that," "Stay with that," or "Notice that" and initiates another BLS set in the same direction. If no change is reported, a different direction of eye movements is attempted (e.g., change from horizontal to diagonal). If no change occurs after two to three different directions, the therapist can switch to another form of BLS and/or use a cognitive interweave, which we discuss later.

The majority of clients will report informational shifts during the interlude periods. Whenever clients do report a change in their experience, the therapist should avoid paraphrasing, interpreting, cognitively refuting, or probing "What do you mean by that" or similar common therapist responses in traditional talk therapy. In EMDR therapy, the intention is to stimulate the dysfunctional information via BLS and allow the client's brain to naturally process the material to its adaptive conclusion. In this sense, the therapist's traditional active-listening, interpretation, and cognitive restructuring behaviors interfere with reprocessing. When therapists do so, they are forcing the client to put distance between their experience to interpret the therapist's question and formulate a response. The therapist does not need to restate or summarize the client's self-report after the BLS because they are aware of their own experience. Therapists should also avoid interfering with the client's experiential state after BLS by exploring the meaning of shifts in memory by asking, "Why do you think that came up?" or "What do you think that means?"

Again, whenever the client reports a change or any new information, their attention should be refocused by saying, "Think of that," "Notice that," or "Go with that," followed by a BLS set. The therapist is watching the client's nonverbal behaviors (e.g., change in breathing, tearing, facial expressions, postural shifts). The actual number of eye movements or time administering BLS will vary according to the client's reactions (F. Shapiro, 2018). Therapists should not rigidly adhere to cycles of 24 back-and-forth movements. The goal is to help clients reach a new plateau as they process information. Sometimes that might result in shorter BLS sets less than 24 and other times, longer sets of 36 to 48 movements.

Associative Processing

The EMDR therapist monitors the client's verbal and nonverbal behaviors for evidence of associative processing. These are the characteristic changes in the client's experiences as reported by shifts in imagery, sounds, appearance (e.g., brighter, bigger, smaller), thoughts, negative statements, insights, sensations, emotions, or positive cognitions (F. Shapiro, 2018).

Whenever a client reports a new emotion (or negative cognition), the therapist should always ask, "Where do you feel it in your body?" with another BLS set. Because emotions can be intense, the therapist reminds the client, "That's it; just remember it's the old stuff." During reprocessing, the client's associative processing (e.g., emotional shifts) can change from sadness, rated as an SUD of 3, to anger, with an increase in SUD to 9. If the client reports feeling "numb" or "empty," the therapist should ask, "Where in your body do you feel that?" followed by a BLS set. The client's physical sensations can change from tightness in the stomach to discomfort in their chest at varying levels of intensity. Images of a perpetrator can become more vivid or start to fade. Negative thoughts of "I'm weak" can shift to "It's my fault" to "I was not responsible." The initial target memory of a sexual assault as an adult can shift to memories of abuse in childhood and memories of supportive relationships.

Client reports of associative processing effects should be followed with "Just stay with that" or "Notice that" and additional BLS sets until the client reports no further changes ("It's the same") and/or reports new positive or adaptive responses ("I survived," "It's over").

Evaluating the End of Phase 4

After each associative link is reprocessed, the therapist is sensitive to reports of new or changing information that is progressively less distressing, and the associations seem to have reached a reasonable stopping point when no new or significant information arises after two sets of eye movements in varying directions. When the client consistently reports positive or adaptive changes, the therapist redirects the client's focus to the original target memory: "Think of the incident [original target memory]. What do you get?" Whatever the client reports, even if positive, it is followed by a BLS set. If the information shifts to negative material, further reprocessing ensues, and the reassessment of the target memory is repeated. At the end of each associative channel, the therapist redirects the client to the original memory.

After retargeting the original (target) memory and completing a BLS set and no new associations are reported (no new emotions, thoughts, sensations, images, etc.), the therapist rechecks the client's SUD level after directing their focus to the target memory: "Go back to the original memory on that scale of 0 to 10, where 0 is no disturbance or neutral, and 10 is the highest disturbance you can imagine. How disturbing does it feel now?" Once clients become familiar with the SUD rating, the therapist only needs to mention, "On that 0-to-10 scale, what do you get now?" When the client reports an SUD of 0, Phase 4 is viewed as complete, and the therapist goes on to the Installation (Phase 5).

Ecological Validity

When the client reports an SUD of more than 0, such as a 1 or 2, and there is no further change reported after the therapist alters the direction of eye movement sets, the therapist asks, "What emotion are you feeling?" Sometimes clients can be confused and give an SUD rating of a positive emotion such as feeling calm or at peace. If so, the therapist redirects the client to provide an SUD rating on negative emotions. If the client continues to report an SUD greater than 0, the therapist asks, "What prevents it from being a zero?" The client's response might indicate a "blocking belief" such as "I don't deserve to be happy" or possibly an ecologically appropriate response such as "My friend died." A blocking belief such as "I don't deserve to be happy" should be considered a new associative channel that is followed by additional BLS sets, and the reassessment is repeated. If the client's response is deemed reasonable or ecologically or culturally appropriate for the client ("My friend died"), the therapist proceeds to the installation phase.

Therapists should not insist that all target memories be reduced to an SUD of 0, but they should be cautious not to prematurely accept a client's statement as appropriate. If there is any uncertainty that the client's higher SUD rating may be due to a blocking belief, the therapist should proceed with two additional BLS sets. If there is no change in the SUD and the client's rationale appears stable, the therapist proceeds to Phase 5.

Blocked Reprocessing

If no movement is reported, therapists should change the direction of the eye movements, the speed of BLS, or increase the length of the BLS set.

Managing Intense Emotional Reprocessing

Some clients (10%–15%) experience an intense emotional release or abreaction during EMDR therapy reprocessing. For some clients, this could be their worst nightmare come true. This is why client preparation has its own phase. In many cases, it is not the client who is overly distressed about their emotional venting but the therapist. Always keep in mind the AIP model. As the client is accessing negative valence memories associated with the maladaptive neural network, some of these experiences had not been metabolized by the brain's information processing mechanism. It may be the nature of the event, who was involved, the degree of dissociation or terror, and/or just random bad luck, but the experience was consolidated in its state-dependent form in implicit, nondeclarative memory, or at least that is what some believe. Nevertheless, this is an event from the past that the client did survive. Moreover, they will get through this again. Therapists need to remind themselves and the client that the reprocessing of these experiences has a beginning, a middle, and an end.

Keeping the foot on the gas pedal (BLS and dual-focused attention), using longer BLS sets, and allowing the brain to reprocess the memory in a more declarative, explicit manner will most likely mean the client will never go through this experience again. Therapists should frequently reassure the client of their presence: "It's okay," "It's just old stuff," "Just notice it," "You're doing fine," "Just observe like scenery through a car or train window," and so forth. The use of a tunnel metaphor can be helpful. Advise clients that "when driving a car through tunnels, most of us feel a little panicky, but keeping the foot on the gas pedal, as opposed to the brake, means we get out of the tunnel sooner." The therapist's presence, dual-focused attention, and longer sets of BLS will get the majority of clients through the tunnel in a few minutes. By keeping calm and reassuring, clients will be able to weather the storm. Look for nonverbal cues or pauses to stop the BLS.

Often, soon after the release of intense emotions, clients' body posture, facial expressions, or breathing rates suggest they hit a plateau, which is usually a good time to stop the BLS and obtain a self-report. If the client's crying makes it difficult to track eye movement, even as the therapist slows down the rate and moves two to three inches side to side, the therapist can suggest switching to vibration, taps, or sounds. Again, when the client and therapist emerge from the tunnel, these can be breakthrough moments (Russell & Figley, 2013).

Strategies for Blocked Reprocessing

We categorize client treatment response to EMDR therapy reprocessing in three broad ways: (a) complete, continuous reprocessing using only the earlier protocol; (b) incomplete or blocked reprocessing due to insufficient access or activation of the negative neural networks (*underresponders*); and (c) incomplete or blocked reprocessing due to excessive access or activation of the negative neural networks (*overresponders*).

Overresponse to EMDR

In my (M. C. R.'s) experience, at least 50% or more clients complete EMDR therapy reprocessing using the basic EMDR therapy reprocessing protocol without any extra intervention by the therapist. Less than 10% of clients demonstrate an *overresponsive* reaction to EMDR therapy reprocessing, characterized by an acute and sustained inability to continue reprocessing by virtue of being overwhelmed by the negative associations emanating from their maladaptive neural nets. Several of the overresponders were on psychiatric inpatient wards, where sufficient safety was afforded to allow reprocessing to continue. Most, if not all, clients who are unable to tolerate the reprocessing effects had an extensive history of early adverse childhood experiences consistent with diagnostic formulations of complex PTSD. The therapist should consider incorporating RDI into the treatment plan before proceeding with additional reprocessing if clients demonstrate a persistent inability and/or unwillingness to continue with reprocessing (Russell & Figley, 2013).

Underresponse or No Response to EMDR

The remaining group of clients, who appear to fall in the *underresponder* category, can receive widely variable treatment courses. For example, some clients may be on track with reprocessing using only the basic protocol, but for some reason, the reprocessing becomes temporarily derailed or blocked. In most scenarios, the therapist can restart the reprocessing by using brief interventions (summarized later). However, a subgroup of underresponsive clients does not seem to respond to reprocessing at the outset. There are a variety of possible, often interrelated reasons clients may report no reprocessing effects, including possible treatment-to-client mismatch, meaning that EMDR is not effective for that particular client. However, before reaching that conclusion, there are a slew of other plausible explanations for client nonresponse, many of which the therapist and/or client have control over and, if identified and resolved, can move reprocessing forward. We have summarized some of the main obstacles for reprocessing in the next section and grouped many into the phases of EMDR treatment where these issues may arise or, if possible, be proactively identified. The attempted solution is often evident by the nature of the problem itself. Often, a client's beliefs, fears, secondary gain, and the like may not be knowable until the reprocessing phase has started. Sometimes it is never known, even when the therapist has inquired. The therapist should pay particular attention to potential therapist variables that can derail reprocessing and seek consultation. The following is our summary of some reasons for non- or underresponding to EMDR therapy reprocessing (Russell & Figley, 2013).

Fear of the Reprocessing. Clients may experience a block in processing due to myriad fears, such as concerns about accessing upsetting information when they have to return to work or go to a special event. Additional concerns might include a fear of losing their competitive fighting edge, fear of the unknown, fear of reliving earlier traumatic experiences, fear of forgetting loved ones, and fear of losing control.

Problems Related to Reprocessing Itself. Other issues that may result in troubles with reprocessing include a mismatch or habituation of the type, speed, direction, and/or length of BLS (e.g., eye movements are too slow and short). Clients who are acutely intoxicated or experiencing sedation from prescribed or illicit substances can have problems reprocessing. Other obstacles include insufficient dual-focused attention (i.e., the client needs greater therapist verbal reassurance), client self-reports exclusively on a single specific target memory component (i.e., after a BLS set, the therapist repeatedly asks, "What happens now with the picture?"), the therapist does not adhere to the treatment plan and does not establish baseline target memories to return to and instead keeps adding new target memories based on the client's week-to-week presentation, presence of a "feeder memory," and the client engaging in metacognition or overanalyzing the EMDR process.

Therapist-Related Factors That Interfere With Reprocessing. A number of therapist behaviors can also contribute to stalled reprocessing—for example, when the therapist is new and/or inexperienced with adhering to the standard EMDR protocol and avoids using an EMDR treatment worksheet, an approach that may confuse both the therapist and client. Moreover, the therapist's disbelief in EMDR theory or treatment or nonadherence to the standard EMDR protocol during the reprocessing phase by overresponding with idiosyncratic or other theoretical methods (e.g., active listening, exploration, interpretation, cognitive disputation) severely limits the benefits of dual-focused attention and BLS, as does the therapist's discomfort with a client's intense emotional reprocessing, fear of their own unprocessed trauma being activated by the client, and engaging in silencing behaviors when the therapist is experiencing compassion fatigue (Russell & Figley, 2013).

Additional Strategies to Manage Reprocessing Issues

Several procedures have been identified to intervene with over- and under-responding clients. There are three options that therapists might use to initiate or restart reprocessing when it seems to be derailed or blocked: (a) change the BLS mechanics; (b) use trigger, image, cognition, emotion, and sensation (TICES) strategies; and (c) use cognitive interweave (F. Shapiro, 2018). Determining which intervention to use depends on where the problem may reside. Generally speaking, starting with the simplest and least invasive is preferred. In this case, the first option for blocked processing is for the therapist to change the BLS mechanics.

Changing BLS Mechanics (Rank Ordered by Preference)

- Solicit client input regarding the angle, speed, width, and distance.
- Check the distance and position of the chairs. Side-by-side "ships passing" is the preferred arrangement. The therapist may be too far from or too close to the client.
- Change the direction or speed of eye movements. Using same the direction and speed may foster stimulus habituation, so try mixing it up.

If using horizontal eye movements, try diagonal movements from the client's lower right quadrant to the upper left. A slower speed leads to quicker habituation and decreases dual focus; try speeding it up. Lengthen or shorten the set; err on the side of longer versus shorter sets. Widen or shorten the width or range.

- Focus on body sensations, especially with cognitively oriented, meta-cognitive clients who report on the process of EMDR versus their material.

- Switch to sounds, vibration pads, or taps (obtain client consent before switching).

- Combine BLS types. Anecdotally, I (M. C. R.) have on a dozen or more occasions combined visual and auditory BLS via an electronic EMDR device for clients when processing appeared to be blocked and/or the client was not responding to any one particular BLS modality or other recommended intervention (i.e., cognitive interweave). Clinically, about 50% of such clients appeared to respond positively to combined BLS by restarting reprocessing. No research has been undertaken to examine the combined use of BLS.

TICES Strategies

TICES strategies contain various ways that the therapist might intentionally alter the client's perception of the image, cognition, emotion, or sensation to heighten or reduce emotional arousal and change the perceptual set in a manner that allows reprocessing to occur (e.g., switching from a color image to black and white or a black and white image to color, viewing a still shot instead of a movie, visualizing the perpetrator without action). Most appear to originate in hypnosis. Therapists are advised to return to the target memory that was altered via TICES and reprocess without distortions. Therapists should tread lightly when considering whether to deliberately distort the client's memory (F. Shapiro, 2018).

Cognitive Interweave

When clients appear stuck in their reprocessing, characterized as reaching a plateau whereby the SUD is not coming down, or they appear to be "looping" or recycling through negative associations without any end in sight, the therapist's initial course of action is always to change the BLS mechanics (see earlier). If that does not work, therapists may use what we refer to as a *cognitive interweave* (F. Shapiro, 2018). A cognitive interweave is an attempt by the therapist to assist the client in accessing and strengthening associations in the client's adaptive neural network. A cognitive interweave is nothing more than a brief comment, statement, image, or question from the therapist containing adaptive information for the client to ponder while BLS is added. Therapists who have used EMDR for a while become accustomed to an extraordinary effect from EMDR therapy reprocessing—namely, the spontaneous, self-generated adaptive statements that clients produce as they move beyond desensitization of disturbance toward personal growth. However, some clients get close but do not quite pull the maladaptive and adaptive networks together. Used judiciously, the therapist's clinical judgment of the client's history and circumstances inform the selection of concise adaptive stimuli for clients to chew on or spit out (Russell & Figley, 2013).

Several forms of cognitive interview have been developed to restart processing:

Education or New Information. Clients may or may not react, but they can be asked by the therapist to "Just think of that." After adding BLS, the therapist can ask, "What comes to mind?" The interweave is designed to enhance the connections between the target memory and the adaptive neural networks.

Other Interweaves.

- "What if your child did it?"
- a metaphor or analogy
- "Let's pretend . . . "
- Socratic questioning
- "I'm confused . . . "
- an atonement metaphor—for example, a reasonable demand or act by the client representing a self-sacrifice or penance that helps others (Silver & Rogers, 2002)

For example, a depressed, demoralized, and defeated junior Marine was blocked in their processing because the client could not forgive themself. The client thought they should have heard their officer's verbal order to move to an adjacent covering during the middle of an intense firefight that resulted in one of the client's squad members being wounded.

Client: If I only had listened to the captain's order to pull back.

Therapist: Wait a minute—I thought you said that you guys were getting slammed by RPGs [rocket propelled grenades] and small arms fire from every direction, it seemed.

Client: Yeah, that's right.

Therapist: Did you talk to anyone in your squad during the firefight?

Client: Absolutely, hard as shit though with all that crap going on; you could scream in someone's ear, and they might not hear you.

Therapist: Sounds chaotic . . . you know the "fog of war"!

Client: Yeah, but if I had done my job right, Smitty would still be here.

Therapist: I'm confused here, Corporal . . . help me understand this: You had to scream in the ear of your squad members right next to you, and they may not have heard everything you said given the chaos. . . . how far away was your captain?

Client: Oh shit, he was on the other side of the road!

Therapist: Think of that. [*Add BLS*]

Client: That's right . . . he was actually about two squads over . . . in fact, I don't remember even seeing him until it was over.

Therapist: Stay with that (Russell & Figley, 2013).

Themes and Cognitive Interweave. Three general themes have been identified that may negatively impact client reprocessing:

- *responsibility.* An adult female was sexually abused as an 8-year-old by her stepfather but has the blocking belief that "It was my fault":

    Therapist: How old were you at the time?

    Client: I was 8.

Therapist: Think of that. [*Add BLS*] What do you get now?

Client: I was only a kid; he was an adult.

Therapist: Stay with that. [*Add BLS*]

- *safety.* A survivor of a violent assault incident 2 years ago is consumed with fear over safety:

  Therapist: What can you do now to make you feel safer?

  Client: Don't get drunk at night and stay with my roommate.

  Therapist: Think of that. [*Add BLS*]

- *choices.* An adolescent was caught shoplifting with schoolmates:

  Therapist: Can you learn from this and make better choices in the future?

  Client: Yes.

  Therapist: Okay, stay with that. [*Add BLS*]

After the client reports the disturbance associated with the target memory as an SUD rating of 0 or higher, if ecologically appropriate, the therapist then goes on to the installation phase.

PHASE 5: INSTALLATION

Admittedly, the term "installation" is an unfortunate choice of words that represents a misleading description of what this critical reprocessing phase of EMDR treatment is about. The therapist does not install anything, but they do aspire to strengthen the client's adaptive information and the previously disturbing target memory. After Phase 4 is complete—with a target memory SUD rating of 0 or 1 (unless otherwise ecologically adaptive)—the therapist proceeds to the installation phase. By doing so, the therapist is attempting to enhance the link between the PC and the target memory. Therapists should anticipate that reprocessing has caused information in the neural networks to shift, thereby the original PC identified in Phase 3 may no longer fit, or another more adaptive PC may have emerged. To check this, the therapist instructs the client to focus on the target memory and says, "How does [*repeat original PC*] sound?" New insights and more adaptive self-statements can result from the reprocessing. For instance, a client who experienced social anxiety with fears of social rejection may have an original PC of "I can learn to relax" and, after reprocessing, endorses a stronger PC of "I am a good person."

After repeating the original desired PC, the client is asked to accept or replace it with a more adaptive one: "Do the words [*repeat PC*] still fit, or is there another positive statement that feels better?" If the client struggles in the moment, the therapist can provide an alternative PC if the client mentioned one during Phase 4. For example, a client involved in a serious motor vehicle accident had an initial PC of "I'm alive," but during the desensitization phase, spontaneously reported a shift in beliefs to "I am a survivor." However, at the time of installation, the client related that the original PC still fit. The therapist queried the client in a manner open to rejection: "You know, at our last meeting, you mentioned something like "I am a survivor." I don't know if that was just in the spur of the moment— is that something you still consider?" The client responded with, "Definitely, I'm definitely a survivor." This became his new PC. It is important that the client, not the therapist, choose the most appropriate PC for themself; the therapist merely assists in the process. If the client accepts the therapist's suggestion, the installation phase proceeds after checking or rechecking (if the original PC is maintained) the truthfulness of the self-statement via the VOC rating (see Chapter 3).

The therapist wants to assess whether the VOC has changed from the assessment phase: "As you think of the incident, how do the words [*repeat PC*] feel, from 1 (*completely false*) to 7 (*completely true*)?" Should the VOC not have increased, the PC is reexamined. An alternative PC should be investigated to find what better fits now. After evaluating the VOC, the PC linkage to the target memory (maladaptive neural network) is intentionally strengthened by asking the client to "Think of the event"—not the original picture because that may have changed—and the client is instructed to "Just think of it" while mentally repeating the PC: "Think of the event, and hold it together with the words [*repeat the PC*]," followed by a BLS set. The

VOC is rechecked with subsequent BLS sets with the target memory and PC linked together until the VOC reaches a 7 (*completely true*). After the initial VOC rating of 7, additional BLS is administered. After the BLS sets, clients are asked, "What do you notice now?" "What do you get now?" If the self-report connotes increasing positive changes and the PC is "stronger" or "more solid," the therapist continues with additional BLS sets until no further change is reported. The reason is that the greater the client's sense of the validity of the PC, the greater the potential for generalization effects and improvements to self-esteem and self-efficacy.

If, after repeated BLS, the PC does not increase to a 7, the therapist explores the possibility of a blocking belief: "What prevents [the PC] from being a 7?" As in Phase 4, the therapist examines whether the VOC level of less than 7 is ecologically appropriate and applies further BLS to the client's rationale to see whether it moves. If not, the therapist proceeds to Phase 6, the body scan. When a dysfunctional or blocking belief emerges that prevents a rise in VOC, the therapist applies BLS sets, and if it does not remit, the blocking belief becomes a new target memory, and the client returns to Phase 4. To ascertain the early memories associated with a blocking belief such as "I don't deserve to be happy," the therapist can ask, "When is the first time you remember feeling this way?" If it is toward the end of the session, the therapist would begin desensitization of the blocking belief in the following meeting due to the likelihood of an emotionally charged memory underlying such negative core beliefs. After the blocking memory is reprocessed during Phases 4 through 6, the therapist will need to recheck the original target memory and complete installation, with a VOC rating of 7 or less, if ecologically appropriate.

PHASE 6: BODY SCAN

Phase 6 is the final EMDR therapy reprocessing phase. The primary goal of body scan reprocessing is twofold: (a) identify and reprocess any residual negative associations in the form of physiological sensations and (b) strengthen the client's connection to their adaptive neural networks. The AIP model informs the EMDR protocol, positing that dysfunctional information in the maladaptive neural networks will invariably lead to somatic sensations linked to traumatic or highly charged memories. Consequently, the body scan is performed by concentrating on bodily tension, pains, or other physical symptoms. After a VOC rating of 7 or less, if ecologically appropriate, and it fails to increase after additional BLS sets, the client is instructed to hold both the target memory and the PC in mind while mentally scanning their entire body from head to toe to identify any residual negative somatic sensations:

> Close your eyes and keep in mind the original (target) memory and the positive cognition [*repeat the final PC used during installation*]. Then bring your attention to the different parts of your body, starting with your head and working downward. Any place you find any tension, tightness, or unusual sensations, tell me.

Should the client report any negative physical sensations, they are followed by additional BLS sets. In many cases, the client will report a progressive reduction in somatic symptoms and a shift to more positive sensations (e.g., "I feel more relaxed"). However, it is not unusual for clients to report an intensification of negative sensations that can be associated with other negative emotions (i.e., fear, anger, sadness, grief) that have existed for a long time but may not have been reprocessed during earlier phases. Sometimes, residual somatic symptoms may reflect a client's unspoken fear of who they would be without their particular affliction or diagnosis. Residual negative body sensations may also be suggestive of accessing a different associated maladaptive neural network.

It cannot be overemphasized how important the body scan phase is in the complete reprocessing of the targeted and associated memories. I (F. S.) recall a female client that I had successfully treated for performance anxiety. When I got to the body scan, she reported a strange sensation in her lower back that she attributed to sitting too long. After targeting the client's back sensation with successive eye movement sets, she abruptly reported a memory that emerged of her being molested by an uncle who held her down on the bed with his hand at the small of her back. The issue of molestation had never been disclosed by the client before and took her aback as well. I then reprocessed the memory of the sexual abuse. Cases such as this highlight the underpinnings of the AIP model that posit that dysfunctional material linked to the presenting complaint of performance anxiety (i.e., the client reported freezing during public presentations) could be associated with the memory of molestation in which they felt enormous distress and anxiety to "perform." Although it was not identified as a problem earlier, this type of antecedent proved to be the underlying cause of an apparently minor presenting complaint. The lesson here is that the therapist should avoid becoming complacent, given the client's presenting issues, and should anticipate that there could be other more significant disturbing material feeding into the present complaint (F. Shapiro, 2018).

Phase 6 is complete after the client, linking in their minds the target memory and the PC, can mentally scan their bodies with no reports of residual negative somatic symptoms. If positive or comfortable sensations are reported, BLS sets should be done to strengthen them until no further change is reported.

Time permitting, the therapist moves on to the next targeted memory per the treatment plan. Or, if this was the last of the past, they move on to the current triggers and then the future template to complete the three-pronged protocol. Due to generalization effects, however, once the earliest and/or worst memory has been reprocessed, the remaining past target memories and the current and future targets have also been reduced significantly in terms of subjective distress measured by the SUD. Therefore, completing the later part of the treatment plan almost invariable proceeds quickly (Russell & Figley, 2013). The next step, Phase 7, provides guidance on how to end a complete or incomplete reprocessing session. Phase 8 describes the procedure for the therapist to check the client's reprocessing between sessions and transition back into reprocessing according to the treatment plan. The client focuses on the target memory and searches for negative physical sensations that, if present, are processed with BLS sets until absent. This provides a check for aspects of the traumatic memory that were not fully processed.

PHASE 7: CLOSURE

During the course of EMDR therapy, a reprocessing session might end due to time constraints after completing the reprocessing of a target memory, though there are other target memories remaining on the treatment plan, or the session might have to be stopped without completing a particular phase for a specific target memory such as reprocessing, installation, or the body scan. Phase 7 provides the therapist with structured guidance on closing both types of sessions and safely preparing clients for transitioning from the reprocessing session back to the here and now.

When Do You Stop EMDR During Treatment Sessions?

Before starting the meeting, the therapist should calculate what time specifically they should be shutting down EMDR therapy reprocessing using one of the following configurations:

- Therapists should finish the EMDR therapy reprocessing within at least 10 minutes (15 minutes maximum) before the end of the 50-minute appointment to allow time for a short debriefing period and a stress-reduction exercise if warranted.
- For 90-minute sessions, leaving the last 15 minutes is adequate for debriefing and a stress-reduction exercise, if needed.

Therapists are encouraged to write down the stop time on a notepad before starting the meeting to prevent confusion at the end.

Looking for Appropriate Times to Finish EMDR

As the session nears the desired stopping time, the following may indicate an appropriate time to start closing the session (Russell & Figley, 2013):

- at a natural pause or plateau after reprocessing,
- when the client reports positive reshifting of information or insight,
- after coming down from an abreaction,

- on completion of the reprocessing phase,
- on completion of the installation phase,
- after a shift to a positive memory, and
- after reevaluating the target memory.

Procedure for Closing a Complete Session

An EMDR therapy reprocessing session is considered complete when the client obtains an SUD rating of 0 (or 1, if ecologically valid), a VOC of 7 (or 6, if ecologically valid), and a clear body scan of any residual negative physical sensations associated with a target memory. About 10 minutes before the end of the 50-minute session, the therapist should advise the client, "We are almost out of time; is it okay to stop here?" Clients are then offered encouragement by the therapist: "You have really done some good work today. How are you feeling?" or words to that effect.

A completed EMDR therapy reprocessing session does not mean completion of treatment, which is determined by reprocessing the three-pronged protocol consisting of all the selected targeted memories in the past, the current triggers, and future template, as well as other disturbing memories in the maladaptive neural network.

Procedure for Closing an Incomplete Session

An incomplete EMDR therapy reprocessing session occurs when the target memory has not been fully reprocessed. This is exemplified by an SUD rating of the target memory above a 1, an incomplete installation phase with a VOC below a 6, or an incomplete body scan that registers on client reports as unpleasant, negative-valenced physical sensations associated with the target memory. When shutting down an incomplete reprocessing session, therapists are recommended to provide the client with sufficient time to debrief with the therapist about their experience in the session. This time also ensures that clients have adequate time to prepare to leave the office safely. The following is a suggested framework for therapists to use for closing down an incomplete session:

1. Respectfully explain to the client, "We are almost out of time; is it okay to stop here?" If, by the odd chance, the client does not respond or communicates that they do not wish to stop, using a sensitive but firm voice, say, "I'm really sorry about that, but we have to end now, and we can pick things up again next week."

2. Reassess the target memory: "Okay, I'd like you to please go back to the memory of [the incident]. . . . What do you notice now?" Write down the client's responses. Obtain an SUD rating: "As you are thinking about [the incident] now, on a scale of 0 to 10, how distressed do you feel now?" Write down the client's response. The therapist should understand that by returning to and reaccessing the target memory, there is a possibility for negative associations to emerge. If that happens, respectfully say, "Okay, . . . well, how about we pick this up again next week? Does that sound all right to you?" There are myriad benefits to this approach:

   - It provides feedback to the client and therapist about treatment progress.
   - It indicates when progress is made, either by a decrease in SUD or new, sometimes adaptive information associated with the target memory; in either case, it may help inspire the client and motivate them to continue.
   - It allows the therapist to record treatment progress in the clinical notes.
   - If little to no progress is reported, the SUD provides input to the therapist to check for possible blocking beliefs; alter the speed, direction, or type of BLS; or implement other midcourse corrections.
   - It offers information on progress or lack of progress to be debriefed at the end of the session.
   - After having the occasional client never return to therapy, call, or answer calls to explain, it seems best to create the opportunity for up-front talk on the client's progress or lack thereof.

3. If the therapist believes the client is too fragile and/or needs to avoid returning to and reaccessing the target memory and the maladaptive neural network to which it is linked, the therapist can ask for a generalized rating of the level of the client's distress without returning

93

to the target memory: "On a scale of 0 to 10, how distressed do you feel now?"

4. Stabilization: If the therapist observes or the client discloses that they are still fixed to negative material, the therapist can redirect the client's attentional focus to the adaptive neural network by implementing a brief stress-reduction technique such as the safe and calm place, combat or tactical breathing, or another containment exercise.

Debriefing the Experience

We developed a script for therapists to use for debriefing clients about the possible residual effects of continued reprocessing effects:

> Processing may continue after our session. You may or may not notice new insights, thoughts, memories, physical sensations, or dreams. Please make a note in your log of whatever you notice. Then do a safe and calm place exercise to rid yourself of the disturbance. We will talk about that at our next session. If you feel it is necessary, call me.

Therapists can develop their own debriefing statement that better suits them and their clients. However, their protocol should preserve the following key messages:

- Reprocessing may continue after the session.
- New memories, feelings, thoughts, insights, and dreams may arise.
- Clients should write down any changes and bring them to the next session.
- Clients, if distressed, can use a stress-reduction technique.
- A safety plan can be reviewed if clients are having dangerous thoughts.

Client Between-Session Logs

Maintaining some kind of log or other self-monitoring tool has been a staple recommendation in EMDR circles for years. For instance, a TICES log consists of six columns, whereby clients document the date of the triggering or upsetting incident, the antecedent or triggering stimuli, and the image, cognition, emotion, and physical sensation, plus an SUD-rating for each notable experience (F. Shapiro, 2018). Therapists are reminded that if they instruct a client to maintain a log of some sort or use another note-taking form (e.g., tracking of nightmares), the therapist should always inquire about the client's log at the beginning of a session. Failure to follow through may communicate that either the task itself was not important or the client's time and effort to comply was inconsequential.

PHASE 8: REEVALUATION

The reevaluation phase of EMDR treatment occurs at the beginning of every EMDR session after the initial meeting. The main purpose is to assess the client's condition in relation to the extent of integration of reprocessed information, as well as check for the emergence of new information that may have been stimulated by the previous reprocessing session. There are essentially four ways the therapist might reevaluate their EMDR work with clients.

Reevaluate Between-Session Changes

- When using this method, therapists might want to consider altering their opening remark by combining their welcoming greeting and initiating the EMDR reevaluation: "What have you noticed since our last session? Has anything changed?" or words to that effect.
- If the client launches into a general review of events from the past week, the therapist should look for the first break or pause and redirect the client's attention to any residual effects from the previous reprocessing session: "Wow, a lot's happened with you. By the way, speaking of happening, what have you noticed after our last EMDR session? Has anything changed?"
- The therapist should note the client's self-report of changes within the memory and new associations, insights, thoughts, images, feelings, and dreams. If clinically salient, the client might include any new associations such as past events, current triggers, or future desired behavior to be added to the treatment plan.

- If it is not the first thing the therapist does, the next thing they should do is ask the client whether they kept a log or wrote down any of their observations since the last session. If so, ask whether it is all right for you to see the client's log (or whatever term they use). If the client is not comfortable with the therapist having the entire log, ask whether the client would read it or a portion of it. If the client is embarrassed or uncomfortable with sharing the log contents—or the more likely scenario that the client did not keep or bring a written record—simply ask, "What have you noticed since our last session? What's changed?"

- One of the important pieces of information that can often be glossed over is whether anyone at the client's work or home or friends had commented about changes in the client or had behaved differently toward the client because of the changes that have occurred.

- Adopting a systems lens, the EMDR therapist might anticipate that if changes are becoming evident in the client's behavior, the client's subsystems (e.g., partner, coworkers, family members) may respond positively or negatively to support or negate those changes. Sometimes, clients harbor ambivalence about their change and the prospects of becoming healthier through therapy. Some may fear that "getting better" may have an unpleasant side effect. Therefore, when clients report observable change(s) in their behavior, it is often fruitful for the therapist to inquire about how others may have responded to those positive changes. Another reason this is an important question during the reevaluation is that it provides the therapist with valuable information about the client's perceived level of social support and recovery environment that we know is vital for sustaining improvement or relapse.

- Once the therapist has reviewed the client's log (if applicable) and inquired about any possible changes that they or others may have noticed since the last meeting, the client is asked to reaccess the target memory in preparation for continued EMDR processing.

Reevaluate the Target Memory From Previous Sessions

- The therapist should be comfortable with rechecking the client's work. If the last meeting resulted in an incomplete session, check the target memory. If the previous session ended as a complete session, meaning the client's SUD was 0, VOC was 7, and the body scan was clear of negative residual symptoms, check the target memory.

- Because of the brain's plasticity and how information can be shifted or reorganized, a therapist always checks whether those adaptive changes have continued or even strengthened or, conversely, whether new negative associations have emerged.

- The therapist could say, "Bring up the incident of _____ that we worked on last session. [Try to name the incident—for example, "mess tent bombing"—to ensure the client is recalling the correct target memory.] What image comes up? What thoughts about it come up? What thoughts about yourself? What emotions? What sensations? On a scale of 0 to 10 [SUD], how disturbing does this memory or trigger feel to you now?"

- To reprocess the target memory from an incomplete session, if the previous session was an "incomplete" session, then on reaccessing and reassessing (using SUD) the target memory, the therapist transitions right into reprocessing the target memory (Phase 4).

Reevaluating the Target Memory From a Complete Session

When reevaluating a targeted memory for completeness of its resolution, all the following are evaluated for any indication of dysfunction.

- The resolution of the primary issue requires an SUD rating of 0, a VOC of 7, and a body scan clear of any residual negative physical sensations.

- Ecological validity is indicated when an SUD of 1 or VOC of 6 is reported and appears valid, given, for example, that the client's combat buddy died and no other blocking beliefs were identified.

- Has associated material been activated that must be addressed? When reaccessing the target memory, any new negative associations need to be reprocessed until resolution.

- Resistance can be dealt with if the therapist suspects the client is still ambivalent about changing their condition; the therapist might ask,

"What would happen if you were successful?" This can be followed by reprocessing.

- Any negative associations that arise in the reevaluation will become the focus of reprocessing before moving on. Continue reprocessing and reassess the original target memory until the target is completely resolved (SUD of 0, VOC of 7, and clear body scan).
- If the client reports that a new current trigger has emerged between sessions and the client asks to reprocess the triggering event instead of an incomplete target from the previous session, the therapist can agree. However, the therapist must ensure the client returns to and reassesses the incomplete target and reprocesses accordingly.
- Reprocessing continues until the completion of the session and, ultimately, the treatment plan.
- The final reevaluation session will occur after completing the treatment plan, which includes the three-pronged protocol of the past, present, and future targets. If the last target memory reveals negative associations have emerged, those are reprocessed until the last target memory is complete on assessment (SUD of 0 or 1, VOC of 7 or 6, and clear body scan). At that time, the client is ready to terminate EMDR treatment.

Terminating EMDR Therapy

Once all the target memories on the EMDR treatment plan via the three-pronged protocol and the positive effects have held at reevaluation, the therapist and client are ready to discuss termination of treatment. To assist the therapist and client in determining the readiness for termination, therapists should review the following four treatment goals.

- Have all the necessary targets been reprocessed to allow the client to feel at peace with the past, empowered in the present, and able to make choices in the future? Has the client been adequately assimilated into a healthy social system?
- Has associated material been activated that must be addressed?

- Have all the necessary targets been reprocessed to allow the client to feel at peace with the past, empowered in the present, and able to make choices in the future?

To accomplish these goals, clients would have reprocessed

- *primary events*—the earliest–worst–recent memories associated with the presenting complaint, usually involving "no more than 20" memories;
- *past events*—negative memories that arise when the client is instructed to concentrate on a particular NC (or NCs);
- *progressions*—any salient, spontaneous negative associations that have emerged during reprocessing that the therapist believes may be contributory;
- *clusters*—reprocessing all identified clusters and rechecking clusters during the reevaluation phase to determine whether any residual associations are present;
- *participants*—clusters of memories associated with a particular person (or persons) that have etiological significance, such as the perpetrator of child abuse or pertinent family members;
- *current triggers*—each processed separately and any new triggers that have emerged, along with any negative past associations that may arise from the client's log or daily report; and
- *future template*—future associations with significant people (i.e., a chance meeting with a perpetrator), anticipatory anxiety associated with future important situations, and integration of adaptive beliefs, mastery behaviors, and self-regulation in the future events question.

The Follow-Up Session

Whenever practicable, it would be prudent to invite the client back after 1 month or so to check whether the treatment effects have been sustained over time. The therapist can repeat the reevaluation steps. In addition to the SUD and VOC baseline measures, therapists should ask the client to complete any previously used standardized symptom measures. If any new negative associations arise, the therapist can discuss with the client targeting those for reprocessing and so on. Should the therapist want to write a case study for a professional article, they should discuss with the client their intentions and how they will protect the client's identity and health care information. When possible, the therapist should obtain the client's consent. The therapist can schedule additional in-person or phone checkups if desired.

Case Illustration

A case example of a client undergoing EMDR therapy is available in Appendix E.

5

Evaluation

In this chapter, we summarize the evidence base of eye movement desensitization and reprocessing (EMDR) therapy and some of the cross-cultural research findings. Psychotherapy research is essentially concerned with three broad questions: (a) determining whether a therapy works in strictly controlled settings (efficacy), especially in comparison with other viable treatments and control groups; (b) determining whether rigidly controlled treatment effects from the laboratory generalize to actual clinical practice (effectiveness); and (c) determining whether a therapy works for the hypothesized reasons (proving the theoretical mechanism of action).

RESEARCH ON EMDR THERAPY EFFICACY

As described in Chapter 2, the history of EMDR therapy is marked by an ongoing debate that continues today over its empirical support.

https://doi.org/10.1037/0000273-005
Eye Movement Desensitization and Reprocessing (EMDR) Therapy, by M. C. Russell and F. Shapiro

Nevertheless, to date, there have been over 36 randomized controlled trials (RCTs) evaluating the efficacy of EMDR therapy with adults with posttraumatic stress disorder (PTSD), nine involving children, and seven regarding acute trauma, along with at least 11 meta-analyses (F. Shapiro et al., 2020). Consequently, the cumulative empirical findings have led to a diverse array of U.S. domestic and international clinical practice guidelines identifying EMDR therapy as a top-tiered evidence-based trauma-focused treatment, including the International Society for Traumatic Stress Studies (ISTSS; Forbes et al., 2020), Department of Veterans Affairs (DVA) and Department of Defense (DoD; 2017), the United Kingdom's National Institute for Clinical Excellence (2018), and the World Health Organization (WHO; 2013) guidelines. Readers will find more detailed descriptions of EMDR therapy research in any of these clinical practice guidelines in Chapter 1 of this book.

In short, EMDR therapy is efficacious in treating a variety of adult trauma-related conditions, including sexual assault (e.g., Rothbaum et al., 2005; F. Shapiro et al., 2020), war (e.g., Carlson et al., 1998; Niroomandi, 2012; Russell et al., 2019), refugee circumstances (e.g., Acarturk et al., 2016; Thompson et al., 2018), natural disasters (e.g., de Roos et al., 2011; Fernandez, 2007), crime (e.g., Harris et al., 2018), terrorism (e.g., Silver et al., 2005), medical trauma (e.g., Haerizadeh et al., 2020), transportation accidents (e.g., Aldahadha et al., 2012; Boccia et al., 2015; Högberg et al., 2008), diagnosis of a life-threatening condition (Arabia et al., 2011; Capezzani et al., 2013; Carletto et al., 2016; Haerizadeh et al., 2020; Osorio et al., 2018), and childhood abuse (e.g., van der Kolk et al., 2007). EMDR is also effective as an early intervention for acute trauma (e.g., Ironson et al., 2021; Nijdam et al., 2012; Scheck et al., 1998).

HEAD-TO-HEAD COMPARISONS

Over the course of 3 decades, EMDR therapy has been compared with a variety of trauma-focused interventions to demonstrate its efficacy. What follows is a brief summary of some of those head-to-head comparisons.

In 1995, Steven Silver and colleagues conducted a large, nonrandomized investigation of EMDR therapy with multiple memories from 83 Vietnam

War veterans diagnosed with combat PTSD. EMDR was found to be superior compared with biofeedback and relaxation training on seven of eight dependent measures, which was impressive but not scientifically rigorous enough to establish efficacy. Subsequently, over 17 RCTs provided head-to-head comparisons between EMDR therapy and other treatment modalities revealing that EMDR therapy effects were at least equal to other evidence-based trauma-informed psychotherapies (F. Shapiro et al., 2020).

An esteemed Cochrane Review meta-analysis reported EMDR and cognitive behavior therapy (CBT) as the two top evidence-based therapies for PTSD (Bisson et al., 2013). Meta-analyses of RCTs with head-to-head comparisons between EMDR and trauma-focused CBT (TF-CBT) found both to be comparably effective (Bisson & Andrew, 2007), with EMDR effects reported as potentially more rapid and efficient because it does not require extensive homework (Seidler & Wagner, 2006). Several trauma-focused clinical practice guidelines concluded that prolonged exposure has generated the most evidence as a top treatment (e.g., APA, 2017a; DVA & DoD, 2017). However, several RCT direct comparisons of prolonged exposure and EMDR therapy reported no significant differences in outcomes (e.g., Ironson et al., 2002; Lee et al., 2002; Power et al., 2002). Moreover, a 2017 meta-analysis of trauma-focused therapies concluded that "PE (prolonged exposure), CPT (cognitive processing therapy) and EMDR were largely indistinguishable as being more effective than one another" (Lenz et al., 2017, p. 349).

Another pertinent study on EMDR efficacy is Barbara Rothbaum et al.'s (2005) research on treating female adults with a history of single incident sexual trauma either in childhood or adulthood (Rothbaum et al., 2005). The research was funded by the National Institute of Mental Health (NIMH). This randomized, well-controlled study involving 74 female rape victims, compared EMDR therapy with prolonged exposure (PE) and a wait-list control. Structured clinical interviews were conducted (i.e., Clinician-Administered PTSD Scale, Structured Clinical Interview for DSM Disorders), and a variety of well-established psychometrics was used to assess depression (Beck Depression Inventory [BDI]), dissociation (Dissociative Experiences Scale-II), and PTSD (e.g., Impact of Event Scale–Revised). All participants received nine treatment sessions. Treatment fidelity for PE and EMDR was assessed by experts selected by Edna Foa and Francine Shapiro, respectively (Rothbaum et al., 2005). Results indicated that both EMDR and PE produced significant treatment effects, with 95% of PE subjects and 75% of EMDR subjects no longer meeting PTSD diagnostic criteria at posttreatment. Symptom improvement was sustained at 6 months, although more of the PE group versus the EMDR group remained completely asymptomatic. This methodologically rigorous, head-to-head comparison met all seven of the RCT "gold standards" (Rothbaum et al., 2005). The significant EMDR treatment effects in this well-controlled study were reported to be contrary to other, less rigorous controlled trials that compared EMDR with cognitive-behavioral treatments (i.e., Devilly & Spence, 1999; Taylor et al., 2003, cited in Rothbaum et al., 2005). In conclusion, Rothbaum stated, "An interesting potential clinical implication is that EMDR seemed to do equally well in the main despite less exposure and no homework. It will be important for future research to explore these issues" (Rothbaum et al., 2005, p. 614).

A 2016 RCT conducted with trauma patients experiencing chronic symptoms of psychosis, depression, and social functioning difficulties compared EMDR, PE, and a wait-list condition and reported both EMDR and PE significantly reduced PTSD and paranoid symptoms and led to remission of psychosis (de Bont et al., 2016). In addition, a blind RCT sponsored by the NIMH comparing EMDR with placebo and Prozac in treating adults with childhood- and adult-onset PTSD found EMDR to be superior to both other conditions (van der Kolk et al., 2007). This would be the last NIMH-sponsored EMDR study. Overall, the results of these head-to-head comparisons indicate that EMDR is at least as effective as other treatment modalities.

EMDR THERAPY RESEARCH WITH
SELECTED POPULATIONS

Combat and War Stress

We covered much of the findings related to EMDR therapy with military populations in Chapter 2. There are books and chapters written on EMDR therapy with active-duty military (Russell & Figley, 2013; Russell et al., 2019) and veterans (Silver & Rogers, 2002) that review the literature and provide specialized EMDR protocols.

To settle claims and counterclaims of improperly researching EMDR in those early RCTs, Carlson et al. (1998) used cutting-edge methods in an EMDR RCT by testing the standard EMDR protocol involving multiple target memories, unlike the previous Veterans Affairs (VA) RCT that focused on a single memory (i.e., Jensen, 1994) and used structured clinical interviews, treatment fidelity ratings, and independent outcome raters. Thirty-five Vietnam War combat veterans diagnosed with PTSD were randomly assigned to receive either 12 sessions of EMDR therapy, biofeedback-assisted relaxation, or routine clinical care as the control condition (Carlson et al., 1998). Researchers reported that 77% of Vietnam combat veterans treated with EMDR no longer met the diagnostic criteria for PTSD at 9-month follow-up. Instead of compelling further research, the 1998 RCT remains the VA's last EMDR investigation, despite identifying EMDR as a top-tier evidence-based therapy for PTSD in the DVA and DoD (2004, 2017) PTSD guidelines. The lack of a single DVA EMDR RCT during the past 20 years of war is a reflection of the harmful scientific bias described earlier (see Chapter 2).

On the active-military side, the absence of any DoD-sponsored EMDR RCT has resulted in circular reasoning by EMDR critics, whereby DVA and DoD leaders cite insufficient RCTs as a rationale to prevent wide-scale clinical training and justify denying treatment access (e.g., Institute of Medicine, 2007; Russell & Friedberg, 2009). Consequently, at present, the only available EMDR therapy research on active-military populations consists of single- and multiple-case studies and large nonrandomized correlational research published by therapists in the field (Russell et al., 2019; see EMDR effectiveness research in the following section).

Complex Trauma

Individuals with severe, chronic, and multiple exposures to adverse childhood events, such as emotional neglect and abuse, especially early in life, are susceptible to developing complex or developmental PTSD. Although not formally recognized in the American Psychiatric Association's (2013)

Diagnostic and Statistical Manual of Mental Disorders (5th ed.; *DSM-5*), the 11th revision of the WHO's (2019) *International Statistical Classification of Diseases and Related Health Problems* has adopted the diagnosis of complex PTSD (CPTSD; Karatzias et al., 2019), and therefore, CPTSD will likely be adopted by subsequent *DSM* revisions. A frequently expressed concern is that trauma-focused treatments may not be safe for individuals experiencing high levels of symptom complexity. To that end, the following overview of EMDR therapy research and CPTSD is offered.

Ehring and colleagues (2014) conducted a meta-analysis of PTSD treatments in adult survivors of childhood abuse. A total of 16 RCTs met the criteria for inclusion in the main analysis that compared trauma-focused treatments such as dialectic behavioral therapy, cognitive processing therapy, emotion-focused therapy, exposure therapy, and EMDR therapy with wait-list and treatment as usual conditions. Results indicated that trauma-focused therapies (including EMDR) were more efficacious than non-trauma-focused interventions and that individual sessions yield larger effect sizes than group treatments.

In 2019, a systematic review and meta-analysis of RCTs of psychotherapies for complex PTSD symptom clusters (i.e., PTSD symptoms, affect dysregulation, negative self-concept, and/or disturbed relationships) was conducted, netting 51 RCTs that met inclusion criteria (Karatzias et al., 2019). Results indicated that EMDR, exposure alone (EA), and CBT were all superior to treatment as usual. EMDR, EA, and CBT had moderate or moderate to large effects on disturbed relationships, and only one EMDR RCT assessed negative self-concept. Overall, few RCTs addressed the impact on affect dysregulation. The authors called for further research on treating CPTSD, including sequencing and treatment delivery (Karatzias et al., 2019).

Therapists contemplating using EMDR to treat clients with CPTSD should extend Phase 2 (preparation) to ensure clients have the capacity to safely tolerate emotional distress linked to their traumatic experiences. Dissociation screening measures should be used (F. Shapiro, 2018). Korn and Leeds (2002) developed a resource development and installation protocol (see Appendix C) to help foster client stabilization and strengthen access to positive emotional states and related coping resources. When the client is capable of remaining present without dissociating or experiencing incapacitating distress, EMDR processing should address the full range of adverse life experiences, including childhood events (F. Shapiro et al., 2020). During processing, therapists are advised to (a) target the client's somatic and verbal responses with bilateral stimulation (BLS); (b) frequently assess for hyper- and hypoarousal, especially dissociation; and (c) be prepared to use EMDR strategies, such as cognitive interweave for blocked processing; while (d) regularly reassuring clients that "It's old stuff; you are in control, and I'm here with you" (F. Shapiro et al., 2020).

EMDR has been identified as an efficient and effective therapy for adults who experienced childhood sexual trauma and adult-onset sexual assault. Indeed, an RCT indicated a 90% elimination of PTSD in rape victims after three 90-minute sessions (Rothbaum, 1997). More recently, van der Kolk and colleagues (2007) conducted a placebo-controlled, double-blind RCT comparing EMDR with Prozac or placebo in treating adults with adult-onset PTSD and adults with child-onset PTSD. Independent raters assessed PTSD symptoms via structured clinical interview (CAPS) and a standardized depression symptom measure (BDI-II). A total of 88 adults diagnosed with PTSD were randomly assigned to each treatment group. At the 6-month follow-up, 75% of the adult-onset PTSD clients (and 33% of adults with childhood-onset PTSD) receiving EMDR saw their PTSD diagnosis enter remission, compared with none of the participants in the Prozac group.

EARLY INTERVENTION

An EMDR protocol for recent critical incidents (EMDR-PRECI) has been developed (see F. Shapiro, 2018) and tested. In all, the 2020 ISTSS meta-analyses (Forbes et al., 2020) examined four studies involving EMDR as an early intervention for diverse traumas (e.g., rocket attacks, factory explosions), resulting in a large significant effect size (SMD = 2.50; F. Shapiro et al., 2020) In another RCT, 17 civilian survivors of a missile attack in a crowded town community were randomly assigned to an EMDR condition using the recent traumatic episode protocol or a wait-list-delayed condition. Participants received EMDR on 2 consecutive days and reported significant improvement on PTSD and somatic symptoms measures that were maintained at 3-month follow-up (E. Shapiro & Laub, 2015).

Moreover, in two RCTs, EMDR was administered in a group format to recently diagnosed cancer patients, resulting in significant symptom reduction compared with those randomly assigned to a no-treatment control condition (Jarero et al., 2018; Osorio et al., 2018). Gil-Jardiné and colleagues (2018) screened emergency room patients for postconcussion syndrome (PCS) and randomly assigned 130 symptomatic individuals to either a 60-minute EMDR session, a 15-minute reassurance group, or a usual care control condition (Gil-Jardiné et al., 2018). The main treatment outcome was the prevalence of PCS and PTSD 3 months after the emergency room visit. Only 18% of the EMDR group went on to report PCS or PTSD symptoms at follow-up, compared with 37% and 65% of participants randomly assigned to the reassurance or control groups, respectively (Gil-Jardiné et al., 2018).

Despite EMDR's potential as an early trauma intervention on military frontlines (e.g., Russell, 2006) and in nonmilitary RCTs, discussed earlier, the relative paucity of RCTs, particularly by the military, and overall small sample size has led organizations like the WHO (2013) to conclude that EMDR's evidence base is emerging.

CHILDREN AND ADOLESCENTS

International guidelines (e.g., Australian Government and National Health and Medical Research Council, 2020; ISTSS [Forbes et al., 2020]; WHO, 2013) strongly recommend EMDR for treatment of children and adolescents with PTSD. EMDR RCTs have demonstrated positive treatment effects compared with wait-list or treatment-as-usual conditions (Ahmad et al., 2007; Chemtob et al., 2002; de Roos et al., 2017). Compared with TF-CBT, EMDR has been found to have equitable efficacy (de Roos et al., 2017; Diehle et al., 2015; Jaberghaderi et al., 2004).

A 2020 meta-analysis examined 16 RCTs in children, adolescents, and young adults (John-Baptiste Bastien et al., 2020). Results indicated a medium pooled effect size for all psychological interventions ($d = -0.44$, 95% CI [-0.68, -0.20]), as well as for TF-CBT and EMDR therapy ($d = -0.30$, 95% CI [-0.58, -0.02]; $d = -0.46$, 95% CI [-0.81, -0.12]), resulting in the conclusions that "EMDR was the psychological intervention that had the greatest effect at reducing PTSD symptoms in children, adolescents, and young adults" (John-Baptiste Bastien et al., 2020; p. 1609), though TF-CBT was reported as the frontline favorite due to the volume of RCTs conducted.

Another more recent meta-analysis systematically reviewed all RCTs since 2017 to evaluate the effectiveness of TF-CBT and EMDR therapy on PTSD symptoms in children and adolescents and assess whether EMDR therapy was effective in improving co-occurring anxious and/or depressive symptoms (Manzoni et al., 2021). Eight studies ($n = 150$) met the inclusion criteria. Preliminary analyses showed that EMDR therapy had comparable efficacy to TF-CBT in reducing PTSD, anxiety symptoms, and depressive symptoms and was superior to the wait-list and placebo conditions. Moreover, EMDR therapy was reported to be more effective than TF-CBT in a shorter period. However, like previous clinical practice guidelines (i.e., WHO, 2013), the small number of EMDR RCTs led the researchers to tentatively conclude that EMDR therapy could be an effective treatment for children and adolescents with PTSD and anxious and/or depressive symptoms. A call for further research is needed to support these results.

EMDR therapy has been demonstrated as appropriate for children of all ages, particularly those who may find PE overwhelming; live in complex, chaotic family systems; and are unable to engage in therapeutic homework tasks (e.g., Gomez, 2013). Like other trauma-focused therapies, EMDR should not be used when children or teens are presently being abused or are experiencing continual exposure to safety threats. The standard EMDR protocol has been successfully used with children with modifications such as alternating puppets to maintain the attention of young children (Adler-Tapia & Settle, 2016). Additional creative and developmentally sensitive variations when using EMDR with children include adopting developmentally appropriate language, using shorter duration BLS sets, using drawings or play materials, and adopting child-oriented modifications of validity of cognition (VOC) and subjective units of disturbance (SUD) ratings (i.e., using pictures; Adler-Tapia & Settle, 2016; Gomez, 2013).

During EMDR therapy reprocessing, creative BLS modifications are used to sustain children's short attention span (e.g., tapping, drumming), including the *butterfly hug*, whereby children wrap their arms around their upper torso and alternate tapping on their backsides or shoulders (F. Shapiro, 2018). In Phase 3, the assessment of negative and positive cognitions may be event specific and present tense and may use feeling-based words (F. Shapiro et al., 2020). Moreover, caregiver responses to their child's traumatic experiences can be a critical factor in recovery; hence, some EMDR researchers have integrated family involvement.

In 2017, de Roos and colleagues conducted an RCT involving 103 children (ages 8–18 years) exposed to a single-event trauma, who were randomly assigned to EMDR, cognitive behavior writing therapy (CBWT), or a wait-list control (de Roos et al., 2017). At posttreatment, 93% of children receiving up to six sessions of EMDR and 90% of CBWT participants no longer met diagnostic criteria for PTSD, with significant reductions on symptom measures of co-occurring anxiety, depression, and behavioral problems, maintained at 3-month follow-up.

Similarly, RCTs investigating EMDR therapy with children (ages 6–10 years) who experienced multiple traumatic experiences (e.g., sexual assault, domestic violence, accidents; Ahmad et al., 2007; Diehle et al., 2015) reported significant treatment effects on PTSD measures after eight sessions (Cohen's d = 0.41 and 0.83, respectively). Diehle et al. (2015) randomly assigned 48 children (ages 8–18 years) with multiple trauma exposures to eight sessions of TF-CBT or EMDR. The primary outcome measure was a structured clinical interview for children and adolescents (CAPS-CA), along with PTSD symptom measures. Both children and their parents reported a significant reduction in posttraumatic stress, depression, and hyperactivity symptoms across treatment groups, with no significant difference in the effect sizes for children who experienced a single- or multiple-event trauma (Diehle et al., 2015).

Finally, Kemp and colleagues (2010) randomly assigned 27 children (ages 6–12 years) experiencing PTSD symptoms following motor vehicle accidents to four EMDR sessions compared with 6-week wait-list controls. An effect for EMDR was identified on primary outcome and process measures, including the Child Post-Traumatic Stress Reaction Index, therapist-rated diagnostic criteria for PTSD, SUD rating, and VOC (Kemp et al., 2010).

RESEARCH ON CO-OCCURRING AND OTHER PSYCHOLOGICAL CONDITIONS

The adaptive information processing model posits that all forms of psychopathology can be explained as dysfunctionally stored information (F. Shapiro, 2018). Therefore, like CBT approaches, EMDR therapy has been studied and shown to be efficacious in treating a wide range of adult psychopathology and other health-related conditions. This is critical due to the fact that comorbidity is common in PTSD (Galatzer-Levy et al., 2013). A recent meta-analysis in research supported by the Taiwan National Science Council included 26 RCTs that found that "EMDR therapy significantly reduces the symptoms of PTSD, depression, anxiety, and subjective distress in PTSD patients" (Chen et al., 2014, p. 1). There is also considerable evidence that EMDR therapy can be an effective treatment for medically unexplained somatic symptoms, including phantom-limb pain (e.g., Rostaminejad et al., 2017; Schneider et al., 2008; van Rood & de Roos, 2009) and chronic pain (Tesarz et al., 2014).

Similarly, another meta-analysis reported large effect sizes of EMDR treatment of co-occurring depressive symptoms along with PTSD (Ho & Lee, 2012). In addition, EMDR therapy has been shown to effectively treat persons with depression, dysfunctional anger, traumatic grief, survivor guilt, and moral injury (e.g., Hase et al., 2018; Meysner et al., 2016). A recent meta-analysis concluded that EMDR therapy is effective with a broad range of anxiety-related disorders, including social or performance anxiety, separation anxiety disorder, panic, and phobias (e.g., Yunitri et al., 2020). It is also effective in treating individuals with substance use disorders, eating disorders, and personality disorders (e.g., Bloomgarden & Calogero, 2008; Brown, & Shapiro, 2006), as well as first responders, healers, and service workers developing compassion stress injuries (e.g., Lansing et al., 2005).

A large RCT examined participants who met the dual diagnosis for psychosis and PTSD who were treated with either PE, EMDR therapy, or treatment as usual. This was the first RCT to investigate the effects of directly targeting the trauma experiences with participants who also met the diagnostic criteria for a psychotic disorder. Despite the severity of the comorbid diagnosis, neither active treatment involved a stabilization phase. Both EMDR and PE led to significant reductions in PTSD symptoms, with a similar effect size to that obtained in studies with PTSD participants without a psychosis disorder (van den Berg et al., 2015). The improvements in social functioning and trauma symptoms were sustained at 1-year follow-up (van den Berg et al., 2018).

However, in 2019, a systematic review of EMDR therapy and the treatment of psychosis included one RCT, two pilot studies, two multiple-case studies, and one single-case report (Adams et al., 2020). Researchers reported that EMDR was associated with reductions in delusional and negative symptoms, with mixed results for hallucinations. In conclusion, the authors wrote, "EMDR appears to be a safe and feasible intervention for people with psychosis. The evidence is currently insufficient to determine the effectiveness," calling for more RCTs (Adams et al., 2020, p. 1).

RESEARCH ON EMDR THERAPY EFFECTIVENESS

R. Bradley et al.'s (2005) meta-analysis on PTSD treatments reaffirmed EMDR therapy's proven efficacy as an evidence-based, trauma-informed therapy but questioned the external validity of all so-called evidence-based treatments for deficient field testing of the effectiveness of these therapies in actual contexts versus artificially controlled laboratory settings that regularly exclude clients with comorbidities. This is a critical observation in light of PTSD research that routinely identifies high levels of comorbidity (50%–80%) with depression, substance abuse, and medically unexplained conditions, to name just a few (i.e., DVA & DoD, 2017).

In short, R. Bradley and colleagues called for future research to shift from unrealistic laboratory environments to actual clinical settings to determine the effectiveness of evidence-based, manualized therapies in clinical practice with a diverse range of clients.

To that end, military clinicians have published small and large EMDR case studies with active-duty patients treated in an array of actual clinical and operational and deployed settings deemed essential to establishing the external validity of evidence-based treatments. Subsequently, EMDR's potential effectiveness was demonstrated at a U.S. Navy field hospital at which four Iraqi war medical evacuees were successfully treated for acute stress disorder or acute PTSD (Russell, 2006), and a U.K. soldier with acute stress reaction was treated at a field mental health unit with sustained improvement at 18 months (Wesson & Gould, 2009). In addition, single-case studies of EMDR treatment in military outpatient clinics involving phantom-limb pain from traumatic amputation (Russell, 2008b), combat-related medically unexplained conditions (Russell, 2008c; Silver et al., 2008), traumatic grief (Wright & Russell, 2013), and inpatient treatment of noncombat PTSD with 40 German soldiers (P. Zimmermann et al., 2007) were all positive, signifying EMDR's utility "in the trenches." Furthermore, a non-DoD-sponsored RCT joint VA–DoD EMDR training program by a handful of military and VA trainers and clinicians monitored training efficacy by conducting a nonrandomized archival chart review of 63 military outpatient treatment cases, including 48 with combat PTSD, submitted by nine military therapists. Significant symptom reduction over an average of four EMDR sessions was reported (eight, if wounded in action; Russell et al., 2007).

In addition, Brickell and colleagues (2015) analyzed archival clinical outcome data from 99 U.S. personnel stationed overseas treated with EMDR at military outpatient clinics and family community counseling centers. Of the 99 archival cases, 65 were active-duty personnel diagnosed with PTSD (42 involved combat, whereas 23 were noncombat related). Across all outcome measures, EMDR treatment resulted in significant clinical improvement (Brickell et al., 2015). Similarly, McLay and colleagues (2016) conducted a record review from 46 U.S. active-duty military members treated with EMDR therapy for PTSD compared with 285 service members with PTSD who did not receive treatment. Results indicated that personnel receiving EMDR therapy had significantly fewer therapy sessions over 10 weeks with a significantly greater reduction of PTSD symptoms than individuals not receiving EMDR (McLay et al., 2016).

Another effectiveness study deploying evidence-based psychotherapy in actual settings was conducted by Hurley (2018), who assigned 30 U.S. soldiers diagnosed with PTSD to two outpatient groups: (a) intensive daily EMDR therapy provided twice a day during a 10-day period and (b) EMDR therapy provided the standard once a week. Results indicated significant treatment gains in both weekly and intensive 10-day formats.

In sum, whether at frontline British combat-stress clinics (Wesson & Gould, 2009), U.S. field evacuation hospitals (Russell, 2006), military outpatient clinics (Brickell et al., 2015; Russell, 2008b, 2008c; Russell et al., 2007; Silver et al., 2008), intensive outpatient treatment centers (Hurley, 2018), military family community counseling centers (Brickell et al., 2015), or German military inpatient hospitals (P. Zimmermann et al., 2007), EMDR therapy has been demonstrated to be a low-cost, highly adaptive, and effective therapeutic tool across actual operational and clinical settings. Nevertheless, much more research on EMDR therapy effectiveness is required, especially with nonmilitary populations.

RESEARCH ON THE HYPOTHESIZED MECHANISM OF ACTION OF EMDR THERAPY

As noted in Chapter 2, while some minor disputes remain over the efficacy of EMDR therapy (i.e., APA, 2017a), by and large, the issue of whether EMDR therapy works has been settled. However, the controversy surrounding EMDR therapy is far from over and has largely shifted to impassioned debate about its hypothesized mechanism of action. Foremost is the question of whether eye movements or other forms of BLS are essential, empirically supported treatment components or merely superfluous, thus designating EMDR as simply another CBT variant

(Novo Navarro et al., 2018; Russell, 2008a). To date, there have been over 30 RCTs that confirm the contribution of bilateral eye movements (Lee & Cuijpers, 2014; F. Shapiro, 2018). In Chapter 3, we reported results of various EMDR dismantling studies investigating BLS and dual-focused attention. A meta-analysis of dismantling studies of EMDR therapy involving both clinical and laboratory settings reported the effect size for the additive effect of eye movements in EMDR therapy as moderate and significant (Cohen's $d = 0.41$), whereas the effect size for the laboratory studies was large and significant ($d = 0.74$; Lee & Cuijpers, 2013).

EMDR THERAPY RESEARCH WITH CULTURALLY DIVERSE POPULATIONS

It is critically important to consider multicultural factors when treating individuals with PTSD or other conditions. EMDR therapists and researchers need to identify what works for whom and under what circumstances in a diverse society. U.S. researchers have recently examined the efficacy of EMDR therapy within culturally diverse populations. For instance, Ironson and colleagues (2021) reported on a sample of 105 predominantly low-income Americans (77.1% African Americans, 11.4% Latinx, and 11.5% other) from the underserved community of Liberty City, Florida, who experienced a traumatic event within the past 6 months (62.1% were violent events, 60.9% involved a death, and 27.6% involved violent death). Participants were randomly assigned to receive four sessions of either EMDR therapy, group stress management with a trauma focus, or group psychological first aid. Results indicated that all groups showed significant declines in PTSD and depression symptoms, but the EMDR group showed the fastest decline, leading the researchers to conclude, "As EMDR gives the fastest relief, it would be the preferred approach" (Ironson et al., 2021, p. 1).

Lipscomb and Ashley (2021) conducted a qualitative thematic analysis of four African American clients interviewed after receiving EMDR therapy. The authors used an antioppressive, critical race perspective to gain insight into the unique treatment nuances, resulting in five recommendations for EMDR therapists working with African American clients:

1. Spend more time providing psychoeducation on the front end. Clarify. What is EMDR and how does it create change? How might clients maintain a level of control while engaging in EMDR? Prepare them for activation in other areas (such as oppression-based memories or experiences) and acknowledge: a) it is a normal part of the process; b) you are able to manage and tolerate these experiences; and c) what they can do if they become uncomfortable or overwhelmed by these memories.

2. Therapist transparency regarding positionality and social location in therapy. How does power and privilege play a role in the treatment process and how does it create barriers and distrust in the work? Who are you as the therapist? How might your privilege become challenging while engaging in trauma work, especially with oppression-based trauma.

3. Create a safer space for client and build a trusting relationship with the therapist. This comes from the consistency in how the therapist shows up in the therapeutic space. Therapists need to build an authentic relationship and foster community prior to starting EMDR with African American clients by inquiring about who they are and incorporating their lived experiences (their histories, their narratives, and ultimately-their strengths) into the therapy space.

4. Therapist must spend more time to get the client use to how this method will impact the client's experience with EMDR (e.g., feeling overwhelmed).

5. Therapist to provide follow up at the end of the session and afterward. Preparation for leaving includes sensitivity to external world and racialized reality. (Lipscomb & Ashley, 2021, pp. 11–12)

EXAMPLES OF EMDR RESEARCH IN THE INTERNATIONAL COMMUNITY

It is not our intent to provide an extensive systematic review of EMDR therapy research outside the United States—that would be another book (e.g., Nickerson, 2017a). What follows is a description of a sample of global studies pertaining to EMDR therapy. For starters, there is a high prevalence of PTSD and its co-occurring conditions reported among refugee and asylum-seeking populations. Thompson and colleagues (2018) conducted a systematic review and meta-analysis of 16 RCTs involving 1,111 participants from Syria, the Balkans, Iraq, Angola, Lebanon, Cambodia, Sudan, Vietnam, Rwanda, Somalia, and Turkey. RCTs were reported for EMDR therapy, narrative exposure therapy (NET), and TF-CBT, including four RCTs using EMDR therapy (Acarturk et al., 2015, 2016; ter Heide et al., 2011, 2016). The authors reported evidence that all trauma-focused psychotherapies were effective but found greatest support for the use of EMDR therapy and NET (Thompson et al., 2018).

Africa

In most sub-Saharan African countries, the burden of traumatic stress is high due to war, natural and man-made disasters, and insufficient mental health resources (Atwoli et al., 2013). Mbazzi and colleagues (2021) reported that since 2007, African social workers, counselors, and psychologists from 13 African countries received training on EMDR therapy by EMDR Humanitarian Assistance Program volunteers from the United States and Europe (see Chapter 2, this volume). Masters et al. (2017) and E. Zimmermann (2014) described their experiences teaching EMDR in Africa. Peters and colleagues (2002) reported the successful treatment of three cancer patients in South Africa. Kane et al. (2015) called for the cultural adaption of the EMDR therapy protocol in Uganda without specific suggestions offered. In Ethiopia, Artigas et al. (2009) developed the EMDR integrative group treatment protocol (EMDR-IGTP), which was tested with 48 Eritrean adolescent refugees, with a reported significant decrease in PTSD and anxiety symptoms (Smyth-Dent et al., 2019). In 2015, the EMDR-IGTP was reported to be used in the Democratic Republic of Congo with 37 young female survivors of sexual assault, compared with individual counseling, with the EMDR group reporting significantly greater symptom reduction (Allon, 2015).

To describe specific cultural adaptations of the EMDR protocol, Mbazzi et al. (2021) solicited feedback from 25 African EMDR therapists (three men and 22 women) representing five African countries (Democratic Republic of Congo, Ethiopia, Kenya, Uganda, and Zimbabwe) who had been using EMDR for an average of 7 years. Therapists described their experience using EMDR. For instance, one Ethiopian therapist reported, "They [the clients] don't want to talk, they say 'wave your hands, it will take away my problems'" (p. 35), and other therapists "described seeing results quickly and feeling EMDR has helped many clients. Clients provide positive feedback and feel relieved; some clients say it is magic, other say 'it's a brain thing'" (p. 35).

Regarding the standard EMDR protocol, most therapists did not use standardized rating scales; in their experience, most clients did not understand the Likert scales, and some felt they were not culturally appropriate. A Ugandan therapist offered the following adaptation of Phase 1 as a more culturally appropriate explanation of EMDR and its use:

> Your brain stores information. When something happens, it creates a memory. You can think of what happened in the past because your brain created a memory. When a bad memory is stored well, it does not disturb you so much anymore after some time. Sometimes it is stored in a bad way, and we need to process that memory again to store it in a better way. You can think of it as a compound with different huts. If the problem is stored in a hut it is safe; if it is still out in the compound, it keeps going around and affects you all the time you cross the compound. In EMDR we want to store your memories in a way that feels safe and does not make you feel bad. (Mbazzi et al., 2021, p. 36)

Cultural Adaptations in the Eight-Phase Standard Protocol

Mbazzi et al. (2021) provided the following summary of EMDR-IGTP adaptations (see Table 5.1). According to these authors, culturally, most clients live together in large households and have shared responsibilities; the therapists explained that just making the client feel better about themselves does not help sufficiently. Clients often have a plural cognition and start with "we are not safe" or "we are bad" because they experience trauma and suffering in close connection to their next of kin (Mbazzi et al., 2021, p. 37).

	Table 5.1	

African Cultural Adaptation to Eye Movement Desensitization and Reprocessing (EMDR) Standard Protocol

Phase	Adaptations
1	Culturally appropriate metaphors of the AIP model
	Use of a visual timeline
	Adaptation and translation of screening tools
2	Put Phase 2 before Phase 1
	Culturally appropriate metaphors to explain EMDR
	Happy or calm place instead of "safe" place
	Basket, bag, pot, pit instead of "container"
	Cultural and religious practices as resources
	Different sign for stop signal
3	Cognition: "We" versus "I"
	Good and bad instead of positive and negative cognition
	Different explanations of emotions
	Adaptation of VOC and SUDS
4	Tapping instead of eye movements
	Include divine powers in cognitive interweaves
5–8	None, other than mentioned above

Note. AIP = adaptive information processing; VOC = validity of cognition; SUDS = subjective units of disturbance. From "Cultural Adaptations of the Standard EMDR Protocol in Five African Countries," by F. B. Mbazzi, A. Dewailly, K. Admasu, Y. Duagani, K. Wamala, A. Vera, D. Bwesigye, and G. Roth, 2021, *Journal of EMDR Practice and Research, 15*(1), p. 36 (https://doi.org/10.1891/EMDR-D-20-00028). Copyright 2021 by Springer. Reprinted with permission.

In regard to BLS type, several therapists described clients as wary of using eye movements, thinking of it as "witchcraft." Other therapists mentioned that using eye movements was fine but that it was better to use a pen or object rather than the hands alone to avoid scaring the client. Most clients preferred tapping as a method. Nevertheless, tapping posed a challenge in some countries where a client cannot be touched by a therapist of a different gender for cultural reasons. Some therapists allowed the clients to do their own tapping by using the butterfly hug for processing (Mbazzi et al., 2021, p. 38).

Cognitive interweaves were also adapted to the reality of clients, with the majority using religious interweaves, as one Kenyan therapist explained: "We often use the presence of God in our interweaves, this helps the client feel there is hope, and they are not alone, it gives them strength" (Mbazzi et al., 2021, p. 38).

In 2020, a group of African EMDR therapists began the process of establishing an EMDR Africa Association similar to professional associations that exist in other continents.

Japan

Masaya Ichii and Ohtsuka (2014) aptly summarized the history of EMDR therapy in Japan as follows:

> The first event in EMDR history in Japan was in 1991. Mark Russell, who was a research associate of Dr. Francine Shapiro visited Japan and taught EMD to us in a small meeting because he married with a Japanese wife. After the Great Hanshin Earthquake in 1995, in July Francine Shapiro attended the first Pan-Pacific brief psychotherapy conference, which was held in Japan. I presented EMD application to the Great Hanshin Earthquake survivors and Francine consulted me. In 1996, we began level 1 & 2 EMDR training with Australian team. Thereafter Dr. Andrew Leeds from California kept coming to Japan for decade. (p. 1)

They continued,

> In 1999, the first special issue on EMDR of professional journal was published. In 2004, Japanese version of Francine's textbook was published. In 2006, the first domestic and academic conference of EMDR was held. In 2008, we began EMDR training with only Japanese team. In 2009, we began publishing Japanese academic journal, which is "Japanese Journal of EMDR Research and Practice." In 2011, we had Tohoku Earthquake and Tsunami Disaster, and we published special issue including 14 articles on helping earthquake and tsunami survivors with EMDR. We visited devastated area, saw ten survivors, utilized RDI for 5 people and applied R-TEP

[Recent Traumatic Episode] protocol to two successfully. Then, we organized EMDR training and consultation group session in marginal area of devastated area. In 2012, kids' book on EMDR was published. In September 2013, 60 minutes TV program, which is exclusively on EMDR was broadcasted by National channel, NHK, and we still receive many telephone calls from audience. (Ichii & Ohtsuka, 2014, p. 1)

Last, in regard to scientific reports on EMDR therapy, they stated the following:

Regarding publications, 118 articles or book chapters on EMDR had been published in Japan by 2012. There have been 64 case studies (56%), 37 introductions (32%), 7 reviews (6%), 7 experiments (6%), 2 supervisions (2%), and 1 investigation (1%). Ratio of sex of case studies population was 25 males (29%) vs. 62 females (72%). Ratio of adults vs. children of population was 60 (69%): 27(31%). Future tasks are considered that controlled trials should be accomplished, database should be made from case studies, and health insurance system, which can cover EMDR treatment, should be established. (Ichii & Ohtsuka, 2014, p. 1).

Indonesia

Susanty and colleagues (2021) designed an RCT protocol that included participants who met the criteria for PTSD and who were receiving public psychological services in Jakarta and Bandung, Indonesia. One hundred and ten participants were randomly assigned to either (a) an eye movement desensitization group ($n = 55$) or (b) a retrieval-only control group ($n = 55$). Participants were assessed at baseline (T0), posttreatment (T1), 1-month follow-up (T2), and 3-month follow-up (T3). Participants were exposed to a script-driven imagery procedure at T0 and T1. The primary outcome was heart rate variability stress reactivity during script-driven imagery. Secondary outcomes included heart rate, pre-ejection period, saliva cortisol levels, PTSD symptoms, neurocognitive functioning, symptoms of anxiety and depression, perceived stress level, and quality of life. Results are pending.

Iran

A number of Iranian EMDR research studies have been conducted demonstrating its effectiveness for a variety of conditions. For example, in an RCT on EMDR therapy for 60 Iranian participants experiencing phantom-limb pain (PLP) following amputation, Rostaminejad and colleagues (2017) reported significant treatment gains in the EMDR group compared with the control group, including a reduction in PLP that was maintained over a 24-month follow-up. Iranian researchers at Yasuj University of Medical Sciences, Iran, described translating the standard EMDR protocol into Persian without other reported modifications, concluding that "this randomized-controlled trial confirm the efficacy of EMDR therapy as an efficient and long-lasting treatment for PLP" (Rostaminejad et al., 2017, p. 213).

In addition, Iranian clinicians reported that 51 Iranian military personnel were admitted to a hospital with the diagnosis of acute combat-related PTSD. Participants were randomly assigned to three groups, EMDR and CBT or a control group, to assess effectiveness as an early intervention to prevent chronic disability. Both EMDR and CBT were reported to be effective in reducing symptoms associated with disturbing memories, anxiety, depression, and anger; however, treatment changes from EMDR were reported to be superior to CBT. The Iranian doctors concluded by recommending EMDR and CBT be used to prevent and reduce symptoms of PTSD in war veterans (Narimani et al., 2008). In a second study, 45 Iranian war veterans diagnosed with combat-related PTSD were randomly assigned to EMDR, CBT, or a control group. Both EMDR and CBT treatment groups had statistically significant pre–post changes on the PTSD Checklist–Military and the Symptom Checklist 90–Revised compared with the control group (Ahmadizadeh et al., 2010).

In another RCT, 14 Iranian girls (ages 12–13 years) who survived sexual abuse were randomly assigned to 12 sessions of CBT or EMDR therapy. Both EMDR and CBT produced a significant reduction in PTSD and behavior problems, but EMDR proved to be significantly more efficient, using approximately half the number of sessions to achieve results (Jaberghaderi et al., 2004).

Last, Iranian medical researchers have conducted RCTs on patients experiencing medical trauma. For instance, Rahimi and colleagues (2019) completed an RCT on EMDR therapy on anxiety and depression symptoms with 90 Iranian medical patients undergoing hemodialysis who were randomly assigned to either a control (no EMDR group) or intervention group (Rahimi et al., 2019). Another Iranian RCT focused on fear of hypoglycemia in Type 2 diabetes, with 72 Iranian patients randomly assigned to EMDR therapy or a no-EMDR control group (Sheikhi et al., 2020). Participants' level of fear of hypoglycemia was assessed before and after treatment with 1- and 3-month follow-ups. The EMDR therapy group reported a significant reduction in fear-related symptoms, leading to the conclusion that "EMDR can be used as a non-pharmaceutical treatment method to treat and alleviate fear of hypoglycemia in type 2 diabetes patients" (Sheikhi et al., 2020, p. 1).

Italy

Fernandez (2007) conducted a field study using standard EMDR therapy for 22 Italian elementary school children (ages 7–11 years) who were buried under a collapsed school that killed a number of classmates during the 2002 Molise, Italy, earthquake. Results indicated significant improvement across measures after an average of 6.5 EMDR therapy sessions. Parents received psychoeducation about trauma and its recovery and attended the EMDR therapy sessions with their child (Fernandez, 2007), which constituted a cultural adaptation of the EMDR protocol.

Mexico

Jarero and colleagues (2105) reported a study involving 25 Mexican survivors of a fatal Mexico City factory explosion who, within 15 days of the traumatic event, were randomly assigned to receive either immediate, wait-list, or delayed EMDR treatment using a recent events protocol (EMDR-PRECI; F. Shapiro, 2018). The EMDR-PRECI group was administered in two 60-minute sessions over 2 consecutive days, resulting in a clinically significant reduction of PTSD symptoms for those receiving EMDR (Jarero et al., 2015).

Republic of Germany

A study compared 40 German soldiers receiving EMDR therapy at a German inpatient facility for non-combat-related PTSD, with 49 German soldiers diagnosed with non-combat-related PTSD receiving group counseling and relaxation training (P. Zimmermann et al., 2007). Greater improvement was reported in the EMDR therapy group. Moreover, 20 soldiers who received EMDR therapy and 14 soldiers who received group and relaxation training were reevaluated after an average of 29 months. Results indicated that soldiers treated with EMDR were significantly improved over the supportive treatment group even after 29 months.

Sri Lanka

Jayatunge (2006), a Sri Lankan military mental health researcher, reported using EMDR therapy on 18 Sri Lankan military personnel diagnosed with combat-related PTSD and found clinically significant pre–post changes on symptom measures. A second case study indicated that large hostile military operations were conducted in Sri Lanka, resulting in a significant number of Sri Lankan soldiers diagnosed with war stress injuries mani-fested as PTSD, depression, somatization, and other adjustment reactions. The author stated that he and other Sri Lankan mental health clinicians received EMDR training in 2005. EMDR treatment of six Sri Lankan soldiers was described. Four soldiers were diagnosed with combat PTSD, and two soldiers were diagnosed with a depressive disorder. After five to eight EMDR sessions, the author described positive treatment effects for PTSD and depression symptoms, with most soldiers becoming symptom free.

Turkey

At least two RCTs have been conducted by Turkish researchers working with Syrian refugees (Acarturk et al., 2016; Yurtsever et al., 2018), along with a pilot study (Acarturk et al., 2015). In all, Syrian refugees receiving EMDR therapy achieved significant improvements compared with a wait-list control; the participants maintained the treatment gains at follow-up, despite living in ongoing unstable conditions (Acarturk et al., 2016).

RESEARCH ON DELIVERY OF EMDR THERAPY AND STABILITY OF CHANGE

A review of the efficacy research on EMDR indicated that for comprehensive treatment of PTSD resulting from a single trauma, the optimal delivery is over approximately 4.5 hours of treatment in 60- to 90-minute sessions (e.g., Marcus et al., 1997, 2004; Rothbaum, 1997; Wilson et al., 1995, 1997). PTSD resulting from multiple traumas may require longer treatment. For instance, an RCT conducted at a Kaiser Permanente hospital (Marcus et al., 1997, 2004) revealed that 100% of single-trauma and 77% of multiple-trauma survivors were no longer diagnosed with PTSD after six 50-minute sessions.

Research on the durability of EMDR treatment effects showed that therapeutic change was maintained up to 15 months after treatment ended (Wilson et al., 1997) and 18 months post-EMDR therapy for adults sexually abused as children (Edmond & Rubin, 2004). Treatment gains following therapy with EMDR are substantial and stable. Loss of PTSD diagnosis has ranged from 48% (Vaughan et al., 1994) to 94% to 95% (Capezzani et al., 2013; Nijdam et al., 2012). When longer term follow-ups have been conducted, improvements after treatment tend to be maintained. For example, the gains in symptom reduction for trauma, depression, and anxiety symptoms at posttreatment were sustained at 18-month follow-up for survivors of childhood sexual abuse treated with EMDR (Edmond & Rubin, 2004). Similarly, trauma symptom reduction and improvements in secondary measures after treatment were maintained at 35-month follow-up for a group of Swedish transport workers with chronic PTSD (Högberg et al., 2008). In the following chapters, we summarize some of the evidence for EMDR therapy with children, adults, and acute traumatic events.

6

Suggestions for Future Developments

Since its 1989 inception, eye movement desensitization and reprocessing (EMDR) therapy has become an extensively researched, effective psychotherapy approach proven to help people recover from trauma and other distressing life experiences. Impassioned debates about EMDR therapy's empirical support have gradually been tempered over the past 3 decades, but the issue is far from resolved. Despite the ongoing controversy, EMDR therapy has rapidly spread across the world. An estimated 200,000 clinicians worldwide have been trained in EMDR therapy (F. Shapiro, 2018). According to the EMDR International Association (EMDRIA), there are over 10,000 trained members. EMDR professional associations exist across Asia, Canada, Europe, Ibero America, the United States, and now, Africa. EMDR Humanitarian Assistance Programs volunteers have provided hundreds of low- or no-cost EMDR trainings and disaster relief services globally. Yet, despite all its achievements, there is

https://doi.org/10.1037/0000273-006
Eye Movement Desensitization and Reprocessing (EMDR) Therapy, by M. C. Russell and F. Shapiro

a great deal more that needs to be done to improve the future reach of EMDR therapy.

MORE RCTs FOR EMDR AND TRAUMA

There is a pressing need for further EMDR randomized controlled trials (RCTs) involving children and adolescents, military, and refugee populations, as well as for EMDR therapy early invention protocols and treatment for complex posttraumatic stress disorder (PTSD) and medical trauma. Ending the harmful bias against EMDR led by U.S. military and veterans' organizations would be a substantial development (Russell, 2008a). Importantly, to date, there have been no dismantling studies of EMDR therapy and other traditional psychotherapies. EMDR has been shown to be at least as efficacious in treating PTSD as mainstream trauma-focused cognitive behavioral therapies even though it violates basic tenets of those exposure- and cognitive-based therapies (e.g., it encourages free association vs. compelling repeated vivid exposure, actively discourages therapist probing or cognitive meaning exploration, disavows detailed client self-disclosure, does not require homework or cognitive restructuring; Russell, 2008a). This is an especially salient question given that vaunted government research agencies such as the Veterans Affairs National Center for PTSD continue to posit that eye movements and other bilateral stimulation (BLS) modalities are ambiguously important components at best or perhaps therapeutically inert, as many EMDR critics assert (U.S. Department of Veterans Affairs, 2020). If true, this should raise serious questions about current treatment procedures and the fundamental principles underlying the traditional evidence-based therapies for PTSD.

MORE RCTs FOR EMDR WITH NON-PTSD RELATED CONDITIONS

As discussed in Chapter 3, the adaptive information processing model provides a broad theoretical framework for conceptualizing not only PTSD but also other forms of psychopathology, similar to cognitive behavior therapy (CBT) models. We are not suggesting that neurodevelopmental conditions such as autism spectrum disorder, intellectual disability, attention-deficit/hyperactivity disorder, or severe psychiatric conditions such as schizophrenia or bipolar disorder are directly treatable by EMDR therapy. However, EMDR therapy research has shown that it can be effective with those populations in terms of processing the experiential contributors (life events) that negatively impact clients' well-being. EMDR advocates are cautioned against overextending claims about EMDR therapy's efficacy in non-trauma-related conditions without adequate empirical support. Doing so has served to perpetuate the resistance toward EMDR therapy (Russell, 2008a).

For instance, specialized EMDR therapy protocols for conditions such as eating disorders have been published (e.g., Luber, 2019), and case studies and quasi-experimental research appear encouraging. It would be a mistake, however, to say that EMDR therapy has been shown to be an efficacious primary therapy for eating disorders, as some authors have appropriately warned (Hudson et al., 1998). Yet, warning against the premature expansion of EMDR therapy is one thing, and stating obvious falsehoods is another—"First, EMDR is sometimes used in conjunction with efforts to 'recover' memories of traumatic events. But 'recovered memory' therapy may carry a risk of inducing potentially harmful false memories" (Hudson et al., 1998, p. 1)—thus perpetuating an unfounded controversy regarding EMDR therapy. A case in point is a thoughtful, systematic review of EMDR therapy for eating disorders that makes the valid point about the paucity of RCTs prohibiting any determination other than that there appears to be promising evidence of EMDR therapy's effectiveness (Balbo et al., 2017). At present, EMDR therapy can be a valuable adjunctive therapy in treating eating disorders (ED), particularly because exposure to traumatic events is a known risk factor for the subsequent development of an eating disorder and has been shown to impact symptom severity in ED clients (e.g., Isomaa et al., 2015).

Additional RCTs are essential to determine whether EMDR therapy may someday be considered an efficacious treatment for ED. The same can be said about EMDR therapy's efficacy in treating other conditions such as substance use disorders, comorbid traumatic brain injury, conduct disorder, obsessive-compulsive disorder, dissociative disorders, medically unexplained physical conditions, phantom-limb and other chronic pain conditions, mood disorders, moral injury, personality disorders, psychosis, traumatic grief, persistent bereavement disorder, posttraumatic anger, and other forms of psychopathology. EMDR therapy RCTs have been conducted on many of these conditions (F. Shapiro, 2018), but declaring efficacy is premature. Research into EMDR therapy's efficacy for persistent complicated bereavement disorder is particularly important because it is included as an official diagnosis in the *International Statistical Classification of Diseases and Related Health Problems* (11th ed.; *ICD-11*; World Health Organization, 2019) and likely in the *Diagnostic and Statistical Manual of Mental Disorders* (5th ed.; *DSM-5*; American Psychiatric Association, 2013) revisions. Future head-to-head comparisons between EMDR and other evidence-based treatments for the aforementioned conditions will also be required to move the field ahead.

MORE RCTs ON EFFECTIVENESS RESEARCH

With efficacy firmly established for all the top-tier evidence-based, trauma-informed therapies, including EMDR therapy, researchers should heed Bradley et al.'s (2005) call to field test these therapies in actual clinical settings (Chapter 5).

MORE RCTs ON THE NEUROSCIENCE OF EMDR THERAPY

There have been over 33 neurophysiological studies conducted on EMDR therapy, including neuroimaging via single-photon emission computed tomography, magnetic resonance imaging (MRI), functional MRI, and near-infrared spectroscopy, that demonstrate functional brain changes occurring during and after EMDR therapy. Greater attention to this important area is needed, especially in the form of RCTs and possible comparisons of EMDR therapy with other evidence-based therapies. In addition, there remains a need for more RCTs into the dismantling of EMDR therapy's two hypothesized mechanisms of action: BLS and dual-focused attention. Similarly, there have been no RCTs to date combining BLS modalities or dismantling the sequencing of the eight phases of EMDR therapy.

MORE RCTs FOR EMDR WITH CULTURALLY DIVERSE GROUPS

In Chapter 5, we reviewed some of the EMDR therapy research available pertaining to culturally based trauma, marginalized groups, and cultural diversity. This remains a critical area in which EMDR therapy (and other psychotherapy) research is sorely lacking.

MORE RCTs ON TELEHEALTH AND EMDR THERAPY

The global pandemic has taught mental health professionals to deliver services via telehealth. A systematic review of EMDR therapy and telehealth was recently conducted (Lenferink et al., 2020); however, only one EMDR non-RCT study was identified and showed "promising results" (Lenferink et al., 2020, p. 1). Whether in response to a pandemic; clients who live in remote, rural areas; single-parent families with small children; or economically disadvantaged or marginalized clients who struggle to get to mental health clinics or offices, there is a tremendous need for investigating the delivery of EMDR therapy via telehealth service.

MORE DISSEMINATION OF EMDR THERAPY

Last, as mentioned in Chapter 2, I (M. C. R.) raised concerns about the merits of accusations against EMDR professional organizations and proprietary practices, particularly as it relates to EMDR training and certifications. With the publication of an EMDR textbook (F. Shapiro, 2018), it was hoped that there would be an opening up of university-based EMDR training in graduate programs similar to other types of psychotherapies. A brief search for university-based offerings finds continuing education with links to EMDRIA-certified trainers versus offerings by faculty. I (M. C. R.) taught a basic EMDR therapy course at Antioch University Seattle as a full-time core faculty member in the PsyD program. However, my trainer status was eventually revoked after I refused to participate in the EMDRIA-approved continuing education requirements required for renewal. At issue was that CBT-oriented professional associations did not require trainer certification or renewal fees or mandate continuing education credits from their organizations.

My doctoral students and I were left with "unapproved" EMDR training, although students could potentially seek EMDR therapist certification via EMDRIA and/or be asked to provide an EMDRIA training certificate by future employers. Although EMDR professional organizations do not strictly forbid the teaching of EMDR therapy at graduate schools— in fact, they tacitly encourage it—it is possible only if faculty have received certified training to be a trainer and periodically renew their certification. According to EMDRIA, graduate students are eligible to apply for EMDR certification as a therapist if they have a graduate degree and are licensed, with an added stipulation:

> Specific EMDR requirements include completion of an EMDR International Association approved training program in EMDR therapy, a minimum of 50 clinical sessions in which EMDR was utilized, and 20 hours of consultation in EMDR by an Approved Consultant. To maintain the credential, EMDR International Association Certified Therapists must complete twelve hours of continuing education in EMDR every two years. (EMDRIA, n.d., para. 1)

The dictionary definition of *proprietary* is "one that possesses, owns, or holds exclusive right to something" (Merriam-Webster, n.d.). By definition, EMDR professional organizations have engaged in and continue to engage in proprietary practices, and as a consequence, they are at least partly responsible for perpetuating the controversy and resistance toward EMDR therapy.

WHERE DO WE GO FROM HERE?
A PROPOSED SOLUTION

To open up the teaching of EMDR therapy across graduate programs and help reduce or end the harmful resistance to EMDR, we strongly recommend that EMDR professional organizations provide faculty members with the EMDR training guidelines and access to training workbooks and allow students of those university-based courses to become certified as therapists, consultants, and so forth. This means lifting the current restrictions that only EMDRIA-approved training is acceptable. Doing so will require a major paradigm shift within the professional EMDR establishment; however, it is past due.

Furthermore, research should be conducted on EMDR therapy training that does not rely on satisfaction surveys of trainees and trainers but includes chart and record reviews as well (e.g., Russell et al., 2007). As reported in Chapter 2, the length of the two-part EMDR therapy training has exponentially grown from 2½ days to 6 days. Aside from anecdotal reports, there is no empirical support for the ever-expanding training requirements that often make EMDR therapy training cost prohibitive for some. There is already evidence that condensing EMDR training to 2½ days was not only practical but subsequent treatment chart reviews also indicated the training was effective (Russell et al., 2007). Undoubtedly, a number of qualified graduate faculty and their students want to teach and learn EMDR therapy in their programs. Removing the current restrictions and barriers and using present credentialed EMDR professionals as sources of supportive collaboration would greatly benefit the field and future of EMDR therapy.

7

Summary

It has been over 32 years since eye movement desensitization and reprocessing (EMDR) therapy was introduced. The overwhelming majority of domestic and international practice guidelines acknowledge EMDR therapy's status as an efficacious evidence-based therapy for traumatic stress injuries, thus offering therapists and their clients a viable, potent alternative to medication and traditional talk therapies (e.g., World Health Organization, 2013). Unfortunately, this has also fueled an ongoing debate or controversy about EMDR that hinders the progression of our knowledge about trauma and its treatment. As discussed earlier, responsibility for perpetuating the resistance to EMDR can be attributed to both detractors and supporters of EMDR: EMDR's harshest critics steadfastly reject the therapy, no matter what the science indicates, and EMDR advocates may overreach the data and/or engage in proprietary actions. We have proposed a solution that will be deemed controversial: opening up the teaching of EMDR therapy in graduate schools.

https://doi.org/10.1037/0000273-007
Eye Movement Desensitization and Reprocessing (EMDR) Therapy, by M. C. Russell and F. Shapiro

As in all psychotherapies, and particularly in trauma-informed approaches, the EMDR practitioner must have good clinical skills, especially in forming an effective therapeutic alliance with the client. However, one of the biggest hurdles therapists face when learning EMDR therapy is that once appropriate trust and rapport have been established, they cannot rely on their previous clinical training while attempting to "do" EMDR therapy. In other words, therapists often find it difficult to dramatically reduce the pull to engage in active listening techniques—exploration, interpretations, and so on—as required in traditional talk therapies. In EMDR therapy, the effective therapist trusts and adheres to the adaptive information processing (AIP) model and standard EMDR protocol. However, adaptations to EMDR protocols may be necessary at times, whether on the frontlines of combat (e.g., Russell, 2006) or to reach culturally diverse populations (e.g., Mbazzi et al., 2021).

Soon after we began teaching EMDR, it became readily apparent that trainees, including many seasoned therapists, benefited from a supervised practicum to learn a novel approach to therapy. A subsequent meta-analysis demonstrated the importance of therapist fidelity to the standard EMDR protocol to achieve the best outcomes (e.g., Maxfield & Hyer, 2002). Appropriate supervised training in EMDR therapy is essential whether such training is provided through professional EMDR organizations like the EMDR International Association or a university.

Globally, EMDR therapy is widely viewed as an efficacious and effective treatment for a broad range of traumatic stressors and populations, and it is increasingly gaining acceptance as a primary treatment for other forms of psychopathology (e.g., Yunitri et al., 2020).

The progress of EMDR therapy over the past 3 decades is a direct testament to the multitudes of dedicated clinicians, researchers, and volunteers. Our sincere hope is that continued rigorous research of EMDR therapy will be undertaken, especially in the aforementioned areas, including neuroscience and cultural diversity, and that doing so may lead to an evolution of trauma-focused therapies like EMDR.

To that end, we believe that future EMDR dismantling studies may uncover new, more efficient ways to reprocess memories that may have people a hundred years from now looking back at the EMDR standard protocol and AIP model in the same way that trepanning (punching holes in the skull to remove bad spirits) is viewed today. If the controversy about and the resistance toward EMDR therapy were to end today, there is no telling what discoveries may lay ahead for a treatment that clearly works but yet violates every major known principle of mainstream trauma-focused psychotherapy. In other words, there is far more that is unknown about the human brain and its workings than is known.

Appendix A:
EMDR Therapy Standard
Protocol Worksheet

Introducing eye movement desensitization and reprocessing (EMDR): The wording of the explanation of EMDR will depend on the client's age, background, experiences, and sophistication.

When a trauma occurs, it seems to get locked in the brain with the original picture, sounds, thoughts, and feelings. The eye movements we use in EMDR seem to unlock the system and allow the brain to process the experience. That may be what is happening in rapid eye movement or dream sleep—the eye movements may help process the unconscious material. It is important to remember that your brain will be doing the healing and that you are the one in control.

PREPARATION

Specific instructions:

> What we will be doing is a simple check on what you are experiencing. I need to know from you exactly what is going on, with as clear feedback as possible. Sometimes things will change, and

sometimes they won't. I'll ask you how you feel from 0 to 10; sometimes it will change, and sometimes it won't. There are no "supposed to's" in this process. So just give as accurate feedback as you can as to what is happening without judging whether it should be happening or not. Just let whatever happens happen. We'll do the eye movements for a while, and then we'll talk about it.

Stop signal: "If at any time you feel you need (or want) to stop for any reason, please raise your hand."

Establishing appropriate distance: "Is this a comfortable distance and speed?"

ASSESSMENT

Presenting issue: "The issue we have agreed to address is _____ _____."

Target memory (or current trigger): "What incident would you like to work on today?" or "The incident we have agreed to work on today is _____."

Image: "What picture best represents the experience to you?" or "What picture represents the worst part of the experience as you think about it now?" If no picture: "When you think of the incident what do you get?"

Negative cognition (NC): "What words go best with that picture that express your negative belief about yourself now?" or "What negative belief about yourself comes up as you think of that picture now?" Have the client make the statement in the form of an "I" statement in the present tense, if possible. This should be a presently held negative self-referencing belief.

Positive cognition (PC): "When you bring up that picture (or experience), what would you like [or prefer] to believe about yourself now instead?" This should be a presently desired self-referencing belief.

Validity of cognition (VOC; for PC only): "When you think of that memory, how true do the words [*repeat the PC*] feel to you now on a scale of 1 to 7, where 1 feels completely false and 7 feels completely true?" VOC = _____

Emotions and feelings: "When you think of the memory the words [*repeat the NC*], what emotion(s)do you feel now?"

Subjective Units of Disturbance Scale (SUDS): "On a scale of 0 to 10, where 0 is no disturbance or neutral and 10 is the highest disturbance you can imagine, how disturbing does it feel to you now?" SUDS =

_____

Location of body sensation: "Where do you feel it (the disturbance) in your body?"

DESENSITIZATION

Initiating reprocessing: "I'd like you to bring up that picture, those negative words [*repeat the NC*] and notice where you are feeling it in your body—and follow my fingers with your eyes."

1. Begin the eye movements slowly. Increase the speed as long as the client can comfortably tolerate the movement.
2. Approximately every 12 movements or when there is an apparent change, comment to the client, "That's it. Good. That's it."
3. It is helpful to make the following comment to the client (especially if they are abreacting): "That's it. It's old stuff. Just notice it." Also, use the speeding train metaphor.
4. After a set of eye movements, instruct the client to "Blank it out" or "Let it go and take a deep breath."
5. Ask, "What comes up now?" or "What are you noticing now?" or "What do you get now?"
6. If the client reports movement or change, say, "Go with that" or "Notice that" (without repeating the client's words) and repeat the bilateral stimulation (BLS) sequence.
7. Going back to the target: When the client's report is neutral or positive for several sets of BLS, ask, "When you go back to the original experience, what do you get now?"

8. When the client reports a SUDS rating of 0, do one more set of BLS; if still 0, proceed to installation. If unable to reach 0, ask, "What keeps it from being a 0?" and follow with BLS.

9. The client should be reporting a 0 or 1 (or otherwise ecologically valid) for the SUDS score before progressing to installation.

INSTALLATION

Linking the desired PC with the original memory or image:

1. "Do the words [*repeat the PC*] still fit, or is there another positive statement you feel would be more suitable?"

2. "Think about the original incident and those words [*repeat the selected PC*], from 1, completely false, to 7, completely true, how true do they feel?"

3. "Hold them together." Lead the client in an eye movement (BLS) set: "On a scale of 1 to 7, how true does that [PC] feel to you now when you think of the original incident?"

4. VOC scale: Measure the VOC score after each BLS set. Even if the client reports a 6 or 7, do eye movements again to strengthen the link, and continue until validity no longer increases. Go on to the body scan.

5. If the client reports a 6 or less, check appropriateness and address blocking belief (if necessary) with additional reprocessing.

BODY SCAN

1. "Close your eyes; concentrate on the incident [or original memory] and the [*repeat the selected PC*], and mentally scan your body. Tell me where you feeling anything."

2. If any sensation is reported, do BLS. If it is a positive or comfortable sensation, do BLS to strengthen the positive feeling. If a sensation of discomfort is reported, reprocess until the discomfort subsides and the client reports a "clear" body scan without negative associations.

CLOSURE (DEBRIEFING THE EXPERIENCE)

"The processing we have done today may continue after the session. You may or may not notice new insights, thoughts, memories, or dreams. If you do, just notice what you are experiencing. Take a snapshot of it (what you are seeing, feelings, thinking, and the trigger), and keep a log. We can work on this new material next time. If you feel it is necessary, call me."

1. After the target memory and trigger(s) are processed, a future template is installed using the following sequence.
2. *Future template*: "We have worked on past experiences relating to your issue, as well as current situations that have triggered you. I'd like to suggest that we now work on how you will respond in the future to the same or similar situations."
3. *Future scene*: "I'd like you to imagine yourself dealing with the same or similar situation in the future, responding in an adaptive way, while thinking of your positive belief [PC]."
4. *Movie*: "Now I'd like you to run a movie with you dealing effectively with this situation, holding in mind the positive belief [PC] you have about yourself."
5. *Challenges*: "I'd like you to think of a challenge situation that could occur."
6. Add BLS to the client's responses until they can visualize coping without negative associations and strengthen the adaptive PC.

REEVALUATION

"Return to the initial target memory and reassess. Bring up the original memory we started with about _____. What happens when you think of the incident now?" or "When you think of the event, what do you get?"

Appendix B:
Safe and Calm Place Exercise Protocol

Step 1: Image. The therapist and client identify an image of a safe place that the client can easily evoke and that creates a personal feeling of peace and safety. For those clients who are unable to feel safe because of the nature of their trauma (e.g., sexual abuse, combat), it is best to identify and focus on a place that allows them to feel calm. If neither of these states is accessible, then identify another positive feeling state (e.g., secure, peaceful, restful, enjoyable):

"I'd like you to think about some place you have been or imagine being that feels very calm or safe. Perhaps being on the beach or sitting by a mountain stream. What image represents your place?"

Step 2: Emotions and sensations. The therapist asks the client to focus on the image, feel the emotions, and identify the location of the pleasing physical sensations.

From *Eye Movement Desensitization and Reprocessing (EMDR) Therapy: Basic Principles, Protocols, and Procedures* (3rd ed., pp. 117–118), by F. Shapiro, 2018, Guilford Press. Copyright 2018 by Francine Shapiro. Reprinted with permission.

"As you think of that safe and calm place, notice what you see, hear, and feel right now. What do you notice?"

Step 3: Enhancement. The therapist may use soothing tones to enhance the imagery and affect. The therapist should take care to convey a sense of safety and security for the client, who is asked to report when they feel the emotions.

"Focus on your safe and calm place—its sights, sounds, smells, and body sensations. Tell me more about what you are noticing."

Step 4: Eye movements. The positive response is further expanded by including a series of eye movements. Rapid bilateral stimulation (BLS) paired with the development of the safe and calm place can occasionally be activating and bring up negative associations. Instead, use slow BLS or omit BLS and proceed through the following procedural steps.

The therapist should say, "Bring up the image of a place that feels peaceful and safe [or calm]. Concentrate on where you feel the pleasant sensations in your body, and allow yourself to enjoy them. Now concentrate on those sensations and follow my fingers with your eyes."

Sets are kept slow and short, four to eight BLS. At the end of the set, the therapist asks, "How do you feel now?" If the client feels better, the therapist should continue the BLS as long as the positive feelings increase. If the client's positive emotions have not increased, the therapist should try tactile BLS or repeat with no BLS until the client reports improvement. If negative feelings come up, identify another safe and calm experience to target.

"Bring up the image of that place. Concentrate on where you feel the pleasant sensations in your body, and allow yourself to enjoy them. Concentrate on those sensations and follow my fingers (BLS set). How do you feel now?"

Step 5: Cue word. The client is asked to identify a single word that fits the picture (e.g., relax, beach, mountain, trees) and rehearse it mentally as pleasant sensations and a sense of emotional security are noticed and enhanced by the therapist's directions. This procedure is repeated four to six times if the positive affect strengthens paired with additional BLS.

"Is there a word or phrase that represents your safe and calm place? Think of ____ [*repeat word*] and notice the positive feelings you have when you think of that word. Concentrate on those sensations and the word _____ and follow my fingers. How do you feel now?" Repeat and enhance positive feelings with BLS several times.

Step 6: Self-cueing. The client is then instructed to repeat the procedure on their own, bringing up the image and the word and experiencing the positive feelings (both emotions and physical sensations) without any BLS. When the client has successfully repeated the exercise independently, the therapist points out how the client can use it to relax during times of stress.

"Now I'd like you to say the word _____ and notice how you feel."

Step 7: Cueing with disturbance. To emphasize the preceding point, the therapist asks the client to bring up a minor annoyance and notice the accompanying negative feelings. The therapist then guides the client through the exercise until the negative feelings dissipate.

"Now imagine a minor annoyance (SUDS = 1–2) and how you feel. Bring up that word _____ and notice any shifts in your body. What did you notice?"

Step 8: Self-cueing with disturbance. The therapist asks the client to bring up a disturbing thought once again and follow the exercise, this time without the therapist's assistance, to its relaxing conclusion.

"I'd like you to think of another mildly annoying incident (SUDS = 2–3), and notice how you feel, then bring up that word _____ by yourself, especially noticing any changes in your body when you focus on your cue word."

Clients are instructed to regularly practice the safe and calm place at home.

Appendix C:
Resource Development and Installation Protocol

RESOURCE DEVELOPMENT AND INSTALLATION PROTOCOL INSTRUCTIONS

1. Identify the needed quality.

   "What quality do you need [more of] as you consider [processing this traumatic experience or meeting this challenge]?" or "How would you like to be able to feel [about yourself] so that you can respond more effectively [in the challenging situation]?"

2. Identify the experience of the resource.

   "Can you remember a time when you personally felt this quality or experienced it when seeing someone or something else?"

3. Identify the image.

   "Describe the experience. [*Pause. Wait for a response.*] What image represents this quality?"

From *Eye Movement Desensitization and Reprocessing (EMDR) Therapy: Basic Principles, Protocols, and Procedures* (3rd ed., pp. 249–250), by F. Shapiro, 2018, Guilford Press. Copyright 2018 by Francine Shapiro. Adapted with permission.

4. Identify emotions and sensations.

   "As you think of that quality or resource, notice what you see, hear, and feel right now. What do you notice?"

5. Enhance the experience.

   "Focus on the position experience. What you see, hear, smell, and notice in your body right now? Take a moment to enjoy your experience. [*Pause*] Tell me more about it."

6. Reinforce the experience of the resource with bilateral stimulation (BLS).

   "Bring up the image of this quality. Notice where you feel those sensations in your body, and allow yourself to experience them fully. Concentrate on the experience and follow my fingers. [*8–10 slow BLS*] How does it feel to you now?"

   If the client reports a positive feeling, image, belief, and/or sensation, the therapist says, "Focus on that [*add BLS set*] What do you notice now?" This is repeated after several slow BLS sets until the resource is strengthened. If the client reports a negative experience, redirect their attention to another experience associated with the resource, or consider another resource (Shapiro, 2018).

7. Identify a cue word.

   "Is there a word or a phrase that represents this resource? Think of [*repeat the word*] and notice the positive feelings you have when you think of that word. Concentrate on those sensations and the word _____ and follow my fingers [*8–10 slow BLS*]. How do you feel now?"

   Repeat with several BLS sets until fully strengthened.

8. Practice self-cueing.

   "Now I would like you to say the word _____ and notice how it feels."

9. Practice future rehearsal using a positive resource.

   "Now imagine the situation that you would like to manage (or respond to) more effectively. Run a movie of your desired response using your resource. What do you notice?"

Add several slow BLS sets until the desired scenario has been firmly established. Length of sets can vary depending on the client's ability to stay with the desired response without activating a negative association.

10. Practice challenging situations (optional).

"Now imagine a challenging situation that could arise. Run a movie of your desired response to this situation using your resource. What do you notice?"

Instruct the client to practice using the resource in situations that are stressful or hard to manage. Evaluate its usefulness in subsequent sessions.

Appendix D:
Sample of Possible Negative and Positive Cognitions

When clients are having difficulty identifying an appropriate negative and/or positive cognition during Phase 3, the therapist can show them the following list and ask them to choose the one that matches their experience the best.

Negative cognitions (NC)	Positive cognitions (PC)
Responsibility and defectiveness	
I'm not good enough.	I am good enough and fine as I am.
I don't deserve love.	I deserve love; I can have love.
I am a bad person.	I am a good (loving) person.
I am incompetent.	I am competent.
I am worthless and inadequate.	I am worthy; I am worthwhile.
I am shameful.	I am honorable.
I am not lovable.	I am lovable.
I deserve only bad things.	I deserve good things.
I am permanently damaged.	I am and can be healthy.
I am ugly, and my body is hateful.	I am fine, attractive, and lovable.

Negative cognitions (NC)	Positive cognitions (PC)
I do not deserve _____.	I can have and deserve _____.
I am stupid and not smart enough.	I am intelligent and able to learn.
I am insignificant and unimportant.	I am significant and important.
I am a disappointment.	I am okay just the way I am.
I deserve to die.	I deserve to live.
I deserve to be miserable.	I deserve to be happy.
I am different; I don't belong.	I am okay as I am.
I have to be perfect (out of inadequacy).	I am fine the way I am.

Responsibility: action

I should have done something.	I did the best I could.
I did something wrong.	I learned and can learn from it.
I should have known better.	I do the best I can, and I can learn.
I am stupid; I am a bad person.	I am fine as I am.
I am inadequate and weak.	I am adequate and strong.

Safety and vulnerability

I cannot trust anyone.	I can choose whom to trust.
I cannot protect myself.	I can learn to protect myself.
I am in danger.	It's over; I am safe now.
I am not safe.	I am safe now.
I am going to die.	I am a survivor.
It's not okay (safe) to feel or show my emotions.	I can safely feel and show my emotions.

Power, control, choice

I am not in control.	I am now in control.
I am powerless and helpless.	I now have choices.
I cannot get what I want.	I can get what I want.
I cannot stand up for myself.	I can make my needs known.
I cannot let it out.	I can choose to let it out.
I cannot be trusted.	I can be trusted.
I cannot trust my judgment.	I can trust my judgment.
I cannot succeed.	I can succeed.
I have to be perfect.	I can be myself and make mistakes.
I can't handle it.	I can handle it.

Appendix E:
EMDR Therapy Case Example

CASE TRANSCRIPT OF THE EMDR
STANDARD PROTOCOL

The client is a 53-year-old married Latinx American, presently employed as a hotel manager and formerly as a police officer. The client identifies as male. He reports being involved in a car accident 3 years ago when a truck ran a light and crashed into the car he was driving with his 8-year-old daughter, killing the truck driver. The client's daughter sustained only minor bruising. The client was referred by the treating psychiatrist for eye movement desensitization and reprocessing (EMDR) therapy because of his deteriorating mental health, despite multiple trials of psychotropic medications (e.g., Prazosin, Celexa, Prozac, the antipsychotic Risperdal) and 4 months of a cognitive behavior therapy approach for "severe PTSD [posttraumatic stress disorder] and depressive condition."

SESSION 1 (90 MINUTES)

Phase 1: Client History

The client was accompanied by his spouse on intake. The client reported being bilingual, though English is the primary language spoken at home. His appearance was disheveled, with his wrinkled shirt partly tucked in, uncombed hair, and unshaven face. According to the client's spouse, the client always took great pride in a clean-cut appearance. The client had a sullen, downcast mood. Responses to the treating therapist's questions were initially terse, requiring the client's worried spouse to fill in the gaps. He complained of daily intrusive images of the truck driver's "bloodied, terrified face" and desperate pleas to "don't let me die!" As the client spoke about the accident, he became tearful. The client's spouse reported he often woke up screaming at night with night sweats. The client has been unable to drive since the incident and is "very jumpy and nervous," especially when riding in the car.

The client also reported, and his spouse confirmed, that he felt excessive guilt and deserved to be punished for not doing more to help the injured driver. The client has avoided going to church, a weekly family routine, and reports no enjoyment in previously fun activities (e.g., playing soccer with the kids). Toward the end of the session, the client's spouse urged him to talk about "the ghost." Eventually, the visibly distraught client reported, "Ever since the accident, I see the driver all the time!" When asked to explain further, the client related that the badly injured driver often appears in the bedroom or bathroom or at other times when he is alone, which is why he tries desperately to avoid being alone. The visions of the deceased driver do not occur only during sleep–wake transitions, nor does the driver ever say anything: "He just stares at me, like he did before." The client denied having any current active hallucinations, delusions, or suicidal ideation.

The main goal of gathering the client's history is to identify the three-pronged protocol, the most salient past, current, and future experiential contributors to the client's psychopathology.

Current Event

The client described the fatal accident memory:

> I was driving home when I saw a truck in my periphery that ran the light. I swerved to avoid hitting him, and the front of his truck clipped me, and I went spinning into a ditch. [*The client reported he did not suffer a closed head injury or loss of consciousness.*] I was in shock about what had just happened and checked myself. My neck hurt, and I was bleeding from my head, but I knew I was going to be okay. I unbuckled my seat belt to find the other driver. I saw his truck was on its side, completely totaled. Somebody, a bystander, came to my car to ask if I was all right, and I told him I was fine but asked about the other driver. He told me that he was hurt really badly and that he had already called 911. When I tried to get out of my car, the bystander tried to stop me, but I told him I was a police officer and needed to check on the driver, so he helped me out of my car, and we walked over to the truck.

He continued,

> Apparently, after striking my car, the driver lost control and ran into a ditch and began rolling. When I went to the driver's side, he was really messed up. Blood was everywhere; he looked in really bad shape. [*Client lowers his head into his hands.*] Me and the other guy tried talking to him to calm him down. He kept yelling that he has a wife and kids and to not let him die. I looked right into his eyes and promised him I wouldn't let him die. Finally, the paramedics arrived and took over. They were working on him after they got him out of the cabin. I saw one paramedic shaking his head. When I walked up to them, they told me, "It's no use, he's already gone."

The client tearfully expressed intense guilt that "I should have done more to save him. I should have avoided hitting him when I saw him . . . I'm responsible for his death!"

Past Events

The therapist asked about other past traumatic events, and the client reported several, including a previous nonfatal motor vehicle accident that he was involved in with his spouse and three children about 5 years ago. The client also reported a memory of responding to a domestic violence call about 8 years ago when he was employed briefly as a police officer. During that incident, the client related that he had allowed an alleged batterer to remain at home and found out 2 days later that the batterer had killed their spouse and 2-year-old son before committing suicide. The client added, "I've lived with that regret ever since." He labeled this memory as the "worst event" in his life.

Last, the therapist asked, "When was the first time you remember feeling this way?" (assessing for earliest onset). The client identified a memory in childhood when left to babysit a 4-year-old sister when the client was around 11 years old. While the client was playing a video game, the sister wandered outside, and the client recalled feeling "panicked, scared, and guilty" when he could not find his sister. The client recalled "looking around for hours" but could not find his sister and had to explain to his mother that the sister could not be found. About 3 hours later, a neighbor escorted the sister back to the family home. This is an example of a *touchstone memory* or possible first experience related to the target memory.

Current Triggers

The client identified driving or riding in a car, being left alone at home, seeing his or other children playing, and sounds of sirens as some of his triggers.

Future Template. When the therapist asked, "How do you see yourself coping with this problem in the future?" the client replied, "I would like to be able to drive again. I need to find a job and support my family." The therapist suggested the goals of being able to calmly ride and drive in a car, and the client agreed.

Treatment options were discussed with the client and his spouse, including using EMDR therapy. The client chose to "try EMDR." The client was asked whether he was comfortable meeting with the therapist alone and consented to do so. The therapist thanked the client's spouse for their invaluable insights and explained that the therapy would likely work best without outside observers.

Phase 2: Preparation (Same Session)

The therapist offered an explanation of the EMDR theory and method:

> Often, when something traumatic happens, it seems to get locked in the nervous system with the original picture, sounds, thoughts, feelings, and so on. Because the experience is locked there, it continues to be triggered whenever a reminder comes up. It can be the basis for a lot of discomfort and sometimes a lot of negative emotions, such as fear and helplessness, that we can't seem to control. These are really the emotions connected with the old experience that are being triggered. The eye movements we use in EMDR seem to unlock the nervous system and allow your brain to process the experience. That may be what is happening in rapid eye movement, or dream, sleep. The eye movements may be involved in processing the unconscious material. The important thing to remember is that your brain will be doing the healing, and you are the one in control.

In addition, the therapist provided the client with a description of what he could expect in EMDR therapy:

> What we will be doing is a simple check on what you are experiencing. I need to know from you what is going on with as clear feedback as possible. Sometimes things will change, and sometimes they won't. I'll ask you how you feel from 0 to 10; sometimes it will change, and sometimes it won't. I may ask if something else comes up; sometimes it will, and sometimes it won't. There are no "supposed to's" in this process. So, just give as accurate feedback as you can as to what's happening without judging whether it should be happening or not. Just let whatever happens happen. We'll do the eye movement for a while, and then we'll talk about it.

Stop Signal

The therapist advised the client, "If at any time you feel you need to stop for any reason, please raise your hand, so I know that you mean for me to stop, and it's not something you're remembering." The client responded, "Okay, I got it."

Demonstrating EMDR Mechanics

The therapist then demonstrated EMDR mechanics by asking the client permission to move the chair beside his "like ships passing in the night." Afterward, the therapist raised their hand in front of the client's face and asked, "Where does it feel most comfortable to have my hand?"; the client settled for about 12 inches from his face. The therapist then demonstrated bilateral stimulation (BLS) using eye movements, starting slowly by moving their hand back and forth laterally, saying, "That's it." When the client's head started turning left to right, the therapist gently responded, "Just track with your eyes only; you can keep your head still." The client acknowledged this and had no difficulty tracking, prompting the therapist to say, "Now I'm going to try to go faster. Tell me if it gets to be uncomfortable for you." The therapist sped up the BLS to the point where the client started having difficulty tracking with his eyes, and the therapist asked, "Is this a comfortable distance and speed?"

Calm and Safe Place Exercise

The therapist then explained to the client,

> The last thing I'd like us to do today is to do something called the calm or safe place exercise. We'll practice using the eye movements. This a technique that people often use to calm themselves down when they get upset after either we do EMDR here in the office or back at home if you get triggered.

The therapist then guided the client through the protocol using the steps described in Appendix B.

The therapist advised the client that he may continue to think about or process the current and past traumatic events discussed that day, and the session ended with the client being instructed to practice the calm and safe place exercise as often as he could and/or needed to. In some cases, it is possible to complete the assessment phase in the first session too, but in this case, the pace of the session was slower than usual. It is also not unusual for EMDR therapy to conform to routine 60-minute appointments and not the optimal 90 minutes.

SESSION 2 (60 MINUTES, 1 WEEK AFTER THE INITIAL SESSION)

After greeting the client, the client related having used the calm place technique several times over the past week: "It seemed to help to distract myself." The therapist then transitioned to returning to EMDR therapy.

Therapist: Last week, we discussed several past memories, including the recent accident, as well as some current triggers, and how you would like to see yourself in the future, right?

Client: Yes.

Therapist: Well, I'm going to ask you specific questions about each of those events. This is the assessment phase for EMDR therapy—is it all right to proceed?

Client: Yeah, let's go for it.

Phase 3: Assessment

Therapist: Okay, last time, you talked about the recent tragic accident when the driver died, and you also mentioned the "worst" experience in your life was that domestic violence incident.

Client: That's right; both are bad because people died, and I was at least partly responsible for it.

Target Memory

Therapist: All right, of those two events, which would you like to start with first?

Client: Probably the car accident because I keep seeing his ghost.

Image

Therapist: What picture best represents the experience to you?

Client: Seeing the truck coming at me, and I tried to swerve to avoid him . . . and seeing the driver pinned against the steering wheel. He was bleeding all over. His face is [a] gray color. He's scared and dying and yells at me, "Don't let me die!"

Therapist: What picture represents the worst part of the experience?

Client: The driver's face, staring at me.

Negative Cognition

Therapist: What words go best with that picture that express your negative belief about yourself now?

Client: I killed him! [While some therapists may probe for a self-referencing belief "I am," the client expressed a lot of emotion, and the guilt is a primary emotion; there are sufficient links for the client to access the target memory.]

Positive Cognition

Therapist: When you bring up that picture, what would you prefer to believe about yourself instead?

Client: I did all I could. I am a good person.

Validity of Cognition

Therapist: When you think of that picture, how true do the words "I can live with what I did" feel to you now on a scale of 1 to 7, where 1 feels completely false and 7 feels completely true?

Client: A 2.

Emotions

Therapist: When you bring up that picture and those words "I am guilty," what emotions do you feel now?

Client: Guilt, shame.

Therapist: On a scale of 0 to 10, where 0 is no disturbance or neutral, and 10 is the highest disturbance you can imagine, how disturbing does the incident feel to you now?

Client: About a 9.

Therapist: Where do you feel it in your body?

Client: I feel tightness in my chest, neck, and shoulders too.

The therapist then went through each of the other target memories solicited during the client history and completed the same assessment. The assessment phase took most of the session, so the client practiced the safe and calm place exercise in the office and was advised to keep using that technique as necessary. The client was advised that EMDR reprocessing would begin the next session.

SESSION 3 (60 MINUTES, 1 WEEK LATER)

After checking in with the client, the therapist reminded him that he had chosen the recent accident as among the "worst" and the first memory to be targeted with EMDR. The client acknowledged that to be true still.

Phase 4: Desensitization

Therapist: I'd like you to bring up that picture of the driver staring at you and those negative words, "I am guilty," and notice where you are feeling it in your body—and follow my fingers with your eyes. [*Initiates set of BLS (about 24 back-and-forth movements)*] What do you get now?

Client: The paramedics came and tried to get him out. I'm telling him he's going to be okay.

Therapist: Notice that. [*Initiates set of BLS as client focuses on what emerged*] What do you get now?

Client: One of the paramedics came over to me and asked if I was the other driver and if I was injured.

Therapist: Stay with that. [*Initiates set of BLS and repeats sequence*]

Client: I watched them use the jaws of life to cut him out. He's not talking or making any noise now.

Therapist: Okay, just notice that. [*Initiates set of BLS*]

Client: As they are treating me and putting me on a gurney, I hear one of the paramedics say, "It's too late, he's gone." [*Client starts crying.*] . . . I can't help to think that I killed him even though I know that it wasn't my fault. He ran the light and crashed into me. . . . I feel tightness in my chest and neck. . . . I started remembering the domestic violence matter and hearing about the wife and kids killed by the guy I should have removed from the home [We can anticipate, according to the adaptive information processing (AIP) model, that the client will free associate to other memories of events that are linked to the original target memory; in response, the therapist restarts BLS without inquiring about the meaning of the event.]

Therapist: Just stay with that. [*Repeats the sequence several times*]

Client: My mind drifted to that earlier accident with my family. [Another example of the client feeling responsible for events that are essentially out of his control]

Therapist: Stay with it and wherever your brain takes you next. [*Repeats the sequence several times*]

Client: Nothing, my mind is blank. It was the other driver's fault. . . . Still nothing, nobody died, and it wasn't my fault. . . . Nothing really.

Therapist: [*After repeated reports of the absence of change*] Okay, let's go back to that original memory of the accident and the thoughts that "I killed him." What do you get now?

Client: I still see his face and get that tightness in the chest. I know it's not rational, but I still do feel some guilt over that. I should have done more to save him.

Therapist: Okay, on that scale of 0 to 10, with 0 being not disturbed anymore and 10 the worst ever, how would you rate that memory now?

Client: Now, maybe a 3 or 4.

Therapist: And where do you feel it in your body?

Client: My neck still and a little tightness in my chest.

Therapist: All right, stay with that and following my hand with your eyes. [*Initiates BLS*]

Therapist: [*During BLS*] That's it—good—it's old stuff. Okay, take a breath. What do you notice now?

Client: I tried to avoid him, but it happened too fast; there was nothing I could do! I feel the tightness in my chest again. . . . When I saw him coming towards me, I thought I was going to die! . . . I feel bad that he died. I tried to help him. I feel terrible for his family. . . . I remember the police officer telling me that there were several eyewitnesses who all said the truck ran the light and that there was nothing I could have done. . . . I remember seeing my wife at the hospital; I was so glad to be alive! . . . I feel lighter now. [*Smiling*]

Therapist: [With BLS] When you go back to that incident, what do you get now?

Client: I'm just glad that I survived but sorry that the other driver did not.

Therapist: [With BLS] When you go back to that incident, if you were to evaluate how disturbing it is to you now, where 0 is neutral—it doesn't bother you at all—and 10 is the most disturbing a person could imagine, what number would you give it now?

Client: It is a 1. It bothers me that the driver died.

Therapist: Think of that. [With BLS] What do you get now?

Client: It's still a 1; somebody died.

Phase 5: Installation

Therapist: When you recall the event, do the words "I did all I could; I am a good person" still fit, or are there other words more suitable you'd like to use?

Client: Kinda, but I think "I survived" is better.

Therapist: Hold the words together "I survived" with the memory of the incident—on a scale of 1 to 7, how true do those words feel to you now?

Client: 6

Therapist: Go with that. [With BLS] What do you get now?

Client: The same.

Therapist: Hold the words together "I survived" with the memory of the incident—on a scale of 1 to 7, how true do those words feel to you now?

Client: I can say now it's a 7.

Phase 6: Body Scan

Therapist: Close your eyes and keep in mind the original incident and the words "I survived." Starting with your head and scanning down to your feet, any place where you notice any tightness, tension, or unusual sensations, just open your eyes and let me know.

Client: No, nothing there. The tightness is gone.

Phase 7: Closure

Therapist: You have done some good work today; how are you feeling?

Client: Much better; I am relaxed. That doesn't bother me now.

Therapist: We are about out of time. As we close today's session, I want to remind you the processing you have done may continue. You may or may not experience new insights, thoughts, memories, dreams, or body sensations. Anything that comes up make a note of it, and we will include it in our next session. You have your safe and calm place exercise, which I want to encourage you to use regularly.

SESSIONS 4 AND 5

Phase 8: Reevaluation

The next session, the therapist instructed the client, "Bring up the original memory we started with about the accident. When you think of the event, what do you get now?" The client reported, "The picture is still faded, but I still feel some tightness in my chest and neck." By the fifth overall EMDR therapy session, the therapist repeated the reprocessing phases until ending with a closure session with similar reports of a subjective units of disturbance (SUD) rating of 0, a validity of cognition (VOC) of 7, and another clean body scan (the term *clean* refers to the absence of any negative somatic sensations).

SUMMARY OF THE TREATMENT COURSE

After reporting no change in the original target memory, with an SUD of 1 and VOC of 7 and adding that he stopped seeing the ghost of the driver, the next "worst" memory was the domestic violence (DV) incident. The initial SUD and VOC of the DV memory taken during Phase 3 revealed an SUD of 9 and a VOC of 2. However, it is quite common in EMDR that the other target memories will likely have been processed simultaneously during the initial target memory, even if they did not emerge during the reprocessing session. When the DV memory was reassessed before reprocessing, the client reported the SUD had decreased to 4, and the VOC had increased to 4. One possible explanation for such changes is offered by the AIP model: Most, if not all, of these highly negatively charged and/or traumatic events are stored and linked together in the maladaptive neural network. Consequently, it is common that the remainder of past target memories is reprocessed quicker than the original target memory. During the fifth session, when reprocessing of the DV murder incident began, the client made several revelations after BLS sets. The client further elaborated during reprocessing that he was on probation as a newly recruited police officer and that the decision to allow the DV perpetrator to remain at home was made by the senior supervisor. Nevertheless, following the DV tragedy, the client left the police force and embarked on a management career.

At the beginning of the sixth EMDR session, the client had been reprocessing the DV memory when he reported that he was surprised to see the driver again. The client related that the driver's face had changed and appeared to have a more sympathetic expression, which caused the client to start to cry and ask for forgiveness. The therapist initiated BLS, and over the course of several sequenced sets, the client reported that the driver "seemed to be nodding and saying goodbye . . . I don't know why, but I get the sense he forgave me, that it was just a tragic accident, and he wants me to live my life and be a good husband and father to my kids." This was followed by several more BLS sets until the DV memory remained at an SUD of 1 and a VOC of 6 because "someone innocent died." This was the last client report of visual hallucinations. The DV memory was reprocessed in two sessions. The client increasingly reported a more adaptive self-appraisal—"It wasn't my fault"—ending with the positive self-statement "I did the best I could."

By the end of Session 8, all the client's past target memories were reprocessed. The therapist then proceeded to the other two prongs of the three-pronged protocol—namely, the current triggers and, once those were reprocessed, the future template. Not surprisingly, the reprocessing of the present triggers and future template was completed quickly (within a single session). A final reevaluation of the original target memory occurred during the tenth and last treatment session. The client reported sleeping better, regaining the ability to drive, and returning to his managerial job. The client also related that being with family was enjoyable again and that he had returned to the routine of going to church weekly. The client and his spouse both expressed the importance of religion in their culture and that returning to church reportedly helped to further resolve some guilt. A follow-up session was scheduled 1 month later, and the client reported sustained improvement.

Glossary of Key Terms

ABREACTION   A normal, potential part of the integrative emotional and cognitive processing of any given target.

ADAPTIVE INFORMATION PROCESSING   Posits a series of interactions and effects involving the centrality of unprocessed memories in conceptualizing and treating a wide range of psychopathology. The concept of an innate psychological self-healing mechanism in the brain–body's information processing system that naturally leads toward an adaptive direction.

AFFECT SCAN   Used when earlier memories are not readily accessible when they occurred at young ages or when clients have difficulty verbalizing negative thoughts or feelings about themselves. It can also be used to get clients unstuck during reprocessing. The client is instructed to hold the target memory and associated emotions while they allow their mind to scan back to an earlier time when they may have felt the emotions.

BILATERAL STIMULATION   Activation of both cerebral hemispheres when tracking rhythmic, alternating, left-to-right stimuli such as eye movements to track visual stimuli (i.e., back-and-forth hand movements or light), listening to alternating sounds, and/or alternating kinesthetic vibrations such as taps or pads.

BLOCKING BELIEFS   Negative self-beliefs that interfere with reprocessing.

COGNITIVE INTERWEAVE   A strategy to change the client's perspectives, somatic responses, and beliefs to the adult or adaptive perspective when reprocessing appears blocked, typically involving three themes: responsibility, safety, and choices.

DUAL-FOCUSED ATTENTION   The simultaneous internal focusing on the traumatic memory or upsetting material coinciding with external focused attention toward an external stimulus (e.g., therapist hand, alternating lights, sounds, kinesthetic sensations).

FEEDER MEMORIES   Untapped earlier memories that contribute to the current dysfunction and block reprocessing.

FLOAT-BACK TECHNIQUE   Used to identify a childhood memory potentially causing current dysfunction that is inaccessible through direct questioning. Clients are asked to think of the disturbing event, identify the negative cognition, notice body sensations, and allow their mind to "float back" to an earlier time and report the first scene (memory) that comes to mind when they felt this way.

NEGATIVE COGNITION   A negative self-statement associated with the targeted event in the present tense. A self-limiting or self-denigrating belief held by the client about their participation in the targeted event.

NODE   The target of EMDR reprocessing that has a pivotal place among the physiologically associated material. When conducting EMDR processing, the client is asked to focus on a target, a specific memory or dream image; a person; an actual, fantasized, or projected event; or some aspect of experience such as body sensation or thought.

POSITIVE COGNITION   A verbalization of the desired state (a self-belief that is a distillation of the positive affect) that is generally a 180-degree shift from the negative cognition.

RESOLUTION   When disturbance is adaptively assimilated through the stimulation of the client's inherent self-healing processes.

TARGET Used to gain access to the dysfunctional memory networks.

THREE-PRONGED PROTOCOL   The assessment strategy of identifying, targeting, and processing (a) the earlier memories causing the problems, (b) the present experiences triggering the disturbance, and (c) the future skills and behaviors needed for adaptive future functioning and to incorporate positive templates for future action.

Suggested Readings
and Resources

EMDR PROFESSIONAL AND TRAINING ORGANIZATIONS

EMDR Asia (https://emdrasia.org). The website links to training in 12 national associations throughout Asia that also help coordinate pro bono training and treatment after disasters.

EMDR Canada (https://www.emdrcanada.org)

EMDR Europe (https://www.emdr-europe.org). The website links to training in 28 national associations. The national associations also provide pro bono training and treatment after domestic disasters. EMDR Europe Humanitarian Assistance Programs provide pro bono training and treatment after international disasters.

EMDR Humanitarian Assistance Programs (https://www.emdrhap.org)

EMDR Iberoamerica (https://www.emdriberoamerica.org)

EMDR Institute (https://www.emdr.com). This website provides general information about EMDR, contact information for EMDR therapists by area, a summary of EMDR research, information on subscribing to a general EMDR Internet discussion list, and order forms for EMDR books.

EMDR International Association (https://www.emdria.org). This website provides training standards and applications to become an approved EMDR trainer and consultant, as well as therapist certification, information on the annual conference and continuing education, and the schedule of EMDRIA-approved workshops. It also lists qualified EMDR therapy training providers throughout the United States.

SUGGESTED READINGS

Abel, N. J., & O'Brien, J. (2014). *Treating addictions with EMDR therapy and the stages of change.* Springer.

Adler-Tapia, R., & Settle, C. (2016). *EMDR and the art of psychotherapy with children: Infants to adolescents treatment manual.* Springer.

Forbes, D., Bisson, J. I., Monson, C. M., & Berliner, L. (2020). *Effective treatments for PTSD: Practice guidelines from the International Society for Traumatic Stress Studies* (3rd ed.). Guilford Press.

Gomez, A. (2013). *EMDR therapy and adjunct approaches with children: Complex trauma, attachment, and dissociation.* Springer.

Knipe, J. (2015). *EMDR toolbox: Theory and treatment of complex PTSD and dissociation.* Springer.

Korn, D. L., Maxfield, L., Smyth, N. J., & Stickgold, R. (2017). *EMDR Fidelity Rating Scale (EFRS).* https://emdrfoundation.org/research-grants/emdr-fidelity-rating-scale/

Leeds, A. M. (2016). *A guide to the standard EMDR therapy protocols for therapists, supervisors, and consultants* (2nd ed.). Springer.

Lipke, H. (1995). *Manual for the teaching of Shapiro's EMDR in the treatment of combat-related PTSD.* EMDR Institute.

Nickerson, M. (2017). *Cultural competence and healing: Culturally based trauma with EMDR therapy.* Springer.

Parnell, L. (2006). *A therapist's guide to EMDR: Tools and techniques for successful treatment.* Norton.

Russell, M. C. (2008). Scientific resistance to research, training and utilization of eye movement desensitization and reprocessing (EMDR) therapy in treating post-war disorders. *Social Science and Medicine, 67*(11), 1737–1746. https://doi.org/10.1016/j.socscimed.2008.09.025

Russell, M. C., & Figley, C. R. (2013). *Treating traumatic stress disorders in military personnel: An EMDR practitioner's guide.* Routledge. https://doi.org/10.4324/9780203829721

Shapiro, F. (2002). *EMDR as an integrative psychotherapy approach: Experts of diverse orientations explore the paradigm prism.* American Psychological Association. https://doi.org/10.1037/10512-000

Shapiro, F. (2018). *Eye movement desensitization and reprocessing (EMDR) therapy: Basic principles, protocols, and procedures* (3rd ed.). Guilford Press.

Silver, S., & Rogers, S. (2002). *Light in the heart of darkness: EMDR and the treatment of war and terrorism survivors.* Norton.

World Health Organization (2013). *Guidelines for the management of conditions specifically related to stress.* https://apps.who.int/iris/bitstream/handle/10665/85119/9789241505406_eng.pdf;jsessionid=F5EB3E2FB9A36EA3B0B150BCA86C454F?sequence=1

PROFESSIONAL JOURNALS

The *Journal of EMDR Practice and Research* (https://connect.springerpub.com/content/sgremdr) is the premier scholarly forum for EMDR practice, principles, and theoretical development.

DEMONSTRATION VIDEOS

Shapiro, F. (Guest Expert). (2007). *EMDR for trauma: Eye movement desensitization and reprocessing* [Film; educational DVD]. American Psychological Association. https://www.apa.org/pubs/videos/4310764

Shapiro, F. (Writer), & Dawkins Productions (Producer). (2006). *EMDR: A closer look* [Film; educational DVD]. Guilford Press.

References

Abel, N. J., & O'Brien, J. (2014). *Treating addictions with EMDR therapy and the stages of change.* Springer.

Acarturk, C., Konuk, E., Cetinkaya, M., Senay, I., Sijbrandij, M., Cuijpers, P., & Aker, T. (2015). EMDR for Syrian refugees with posttraumatic stress disorder symptoms: Results of a pilot randomized controlled trial. *European Journal of Psychotraumatology, 6*(1), 27414. https://doi.org/10.3402/ejpt.v6.27414

Acarturk, C., Konuk, E., Cetinkaya, M., Senay, I., Sijbrandij, M., Gulen, B., & Cuijpers, P. (2016). The efficacy of eye movement desensitization and reprocessing for post-traumatic stress disorder and depression among Syrian refugees: Results of a randomized controlled trial. *Psychological Medicine, 46*(12), 2583–2593. https://doi.org/10.1017/S0033291716001070

Adams, R., Ohlsen, S., & Wood, E. (2020). Eye movement desensitization and reprocessing (EMDR) for the treatment of psychosis: A systematic review. *European Journal of Psychotraumatology, 11*(1), 1711349. https://doi.org/10.1080/20008198.2019.1711349

Adler-Tapia, R., & Settle, C. (2016). *EMDR and the art of psychotherapy with children: Infants to adolescents treatment manual.* Springer.

Ahmad, A., Larsson, B., & Sundelin-Wahlsten, V. (2007). EMDR treatment for children with PTSD: Results of a randomized controlled trial. *Nordic Journal of Psychiatry, 61*(5), 349–354. https://doi.org/10.1080/08039480701643464

Ahmadizadeh M. J., Eskandari H., Falsafinejad M. R., & Borjali A. (2010). Comparison of the effectiveness of cognitive-behavioral and eye movement desensitization reprocessing treatment models on patients with war post-traumatic stress disorder. *Iranian Journal of Military Medicine, 12*(3), 173–178.

Aldahadha, B., Harthy, H. A., & Sulaiman, S. (2012). The efficacy of eye movement desensitization reprocessing in resolving the trauma caused by the road accidents in the Sultanate of Oman. *Journal of Instructional Psychology, 39,* 146–159.

Allon, M. (2015). EMDR group therapy with women who were sexually assaulted in the Congo. *Journal of EMDR Practice and Research, 9*(1), 28–34. https://doi.org/10.1891/1933-3196.9.1.28

American Psychiatric Association. (1980). *Diagnostic and statistical manual of mental disorders* (3rd ed.). American Psychiatric Association.

American Psychiatric Association. (2013). *Diagnostic and statistical manual of mental disorders* (5th ed.). American Psychiatric Association.

American Psychological Association. (2017a). *Clinical practice guideline for the treatment of posttraumatic stress disorder (PTSD) in adults.* https://www.apa.org/ptsd-guideline

American Psychological Association. (2017b). *Ethical principles of psychologists and code of conduct* (2002, amended effective June 1, 2010, and January 1, 2017). https://www.apa.org/ethics/code/index.aspx

Arabia, E., Manca, M. L., & Solomon, R. M. (2011). EMDR for survivors of life-threatening cardiac events: Results of a pilot study. *Journal of EMDR Practice and Research, 5*(1), 2–13. https://doi.org/10.1891/1933-3196.5.1.2

Artigas, L., Jarero, I., Alcala, N., & Cano, T. L. (2009). The EMDR integrative group treatment protocol (IGTP). In M. Luber (Ed.), *Eye movement desensitization and reprocessing (EMDR) scripted protocols: Basics and special situations* (pp. 279–288). Springer.

Atwoli, L., Stein, D. J., Williams, D. R., Mclaughlin, K. A., Petukhova, M., Kessler, R. C., & Koenen, K. C. (2013). Trauma and posttraumatic stress disorder in South Africa: Analysis from the South African Stress and Health Study. *BMC Psychiatry, 13*(1), 182. https://doi.org/10.1186/1471-244X-13-182

Australian Government and National Health and Medical Research Council. (2020). *Australian guidelines for the prevention and treatment of acute stress disorder, posttraumatic stress disorder, and complex PTSD.* Australian Centre for Posttraumatic Mental Health. https://www.phoenixaustralia.org/australian-guidelines-for-ptsd/

Baddeley, A. (2012). Working memory: Theories, models, and controversies. *Annual Review of Psychology, 63*(1), 1–29. https://doi.org/10.1146/annurev-psych-120710-100422

Balbo, M., Zaccagnino, M., Cussino, M., & Civiiotti, C. (2017). Eye movement desensitization and reprocessing (EMDR) and eating disorders: A systematic review. *Clinical Neuropsychiatry: Journal of Treatment Evaluation, 14*(5), 321–329.

Barrowcliff, A. L., Gray, N. S., Freeman, T. C. A., & MacCulloch, M. J. (2004). Eye movements reduce the vividness, emotional valence, and electrodermal arousal associated with negative autobiographical memories. *Journal of Forensic Psychiatry & Psychology*, 15(2), 325–345. https://doi.org/10.1080/14789940410001673042

Baskin, T. W., Tierney, S. C., Minami, T., & Wampold, B. E. (2003). Establishing specificity in psychotherapy: A meta-analysis of structural equivalence of placebo controls. *Journal of Consulting and Clinical Psychology*, 71(6), 973–979. https://doi.org/10.1037/0022-006X.71.6.973

Bisson, J., & Andrew, M. (2007). Psychological treatment of posttraumatic stress disorder (PTSD). *Cochrane Database of Systematic Reviews*. https://doi.org/10.1002/14651858.CD003388.pub3

Bloomgarden, A., & Calogero, R. M. (2008). A randomized experimental test of the efficacy of EMDR treatment on negative body image in eating disorder inpatients. *Eating Disorders*, 16(5), 418–427. https://doi.org/10.1080/10640260802370598

Boccia, M., Piccardi, L., Cordellieri, P., Guariglia, C., & Giannini, A. M. (2015). EMDR therapy for PTSD after motor vehicle accidents: Meta-analytic evidence for specific treatment. *Frontiers in Human Neuroscience*, 9, 1–9. https://doi.org/10.3389/fnhum.2015.00213

Bossini, L., Santarnecchi, E., Casolaro, I., Koukouna, D., Caterini, C., Cecchini, F., Fortini, V., Vatti, G., Marino, D., Fernandez, I., Rossi, A., & Fagiolini, A. (2017). Morphovolumetric changes after EMDR treatment in drug-naïve PTSD patients. *Rivista di Psichiatria*, 52(1), 24–31.

Boudewyns, P. A., & Hyer, L. A. (1996). Eye movement desensitization and reprocessing (EMDR) as treatment for post-traumatic stress disorder (PTSD). *Clinical Psychology & Psychotherapy*, 3(3), 185–195. https://doi.org/10.1002/(SICI)1099-0879(199609)3:3<185::AID-CPP101>3.0.CO;2-0

Boukezzi, S., El Khoury-Malhame, M., Auzias, G., Reynaud, E., Rousseau, P. F., Richard, E., Zendjidjian, X., Roques, J., Castelli, N., Correard, N., Guyon, V., Gellato, C., Samuelian, J. C., Cancel, A., Comte, M., Latinus, M., Guedj, E., & Khalfa, S. (2017). Grey matter density changes of structures involved in posttraumatic stress disorder (PTSD) after recovery following eye movement desensitization and reprocessing (EMDR) therapy. *Psychiatry Research: Neuroimaging*, 266, 146–152. https://doi.org/10.1016/j.pscychresns.2017.06.009

Bradley, M. M. (2009). Natural selective attention: Orienting and emotion. *Psychophysiology*, 46(1), 1–11. https://doi.org/10.1111/j.1469-8986.2008.00702.x

Bradley, R., Greene, J., Russ, E., Dutra, L., & Westen, D. (2005). A multidimensional meta-analysis of psychotherapy for PTSD. *The American Journal of Psychiatry*, 162(2), 214–227. https://doi.org/10.1176/appi.ajp.162.2.214

Brickell, M., Russell, M. C., & Smith, R. (2015). The effectiveness of evidence-based treatments of active military personnel and their families. *Journal of EMDR Theory and Practice*, 9(4), 198–208. https://doi.org/10.1891/1933-3196.9.4.198

Brown, S., & Shapiro, F. (2006). EMDR in the treatment of borderline personality disorder. *Clinical Case Studies, 5*(5), 403–420. https://doi.org/10.1177/1534650104271773

Capezzani, L., Ostacoli, L., Cavallo, M., Carletoo, S., Fernandez, I., Solomon, R., Pagani, M., & Cantelmi, T. (2013). EMDR and CBT for cancer patients: Comparative study of effects on PTSD, anxiety, and depression. *Journal of EMDR Practice and Research, 7*(3), 134–143. https://doi.org/10.1891/1933-3196.7.3.134

Carletto, S., Borghi, M., Bertino, G., Oliva, F., Cavallo, M., Hofmann, A., Zennaro, A., Malucchi, S., & Ostacoli, L. (2016). Treating post-traumatic stress disorder in patients with multiple sclerosis: A randomized controlled trial comparing the efficacy of eye movement desensitization and reprocessing and relaxation therapy. *Frontiers in Psychology, 7*, 526. https://doi.org/10.3389/fpsyg.2016.00526

Carlson, J. G., Chemtob, C. M., Rusnak, K., Hedlund, N. L., & Muraoka, M. Y. (1998). Eye movement desensitization and reprocessing (EDMR) treatment for combat-related posttraumatic stress disorder. *Journal of Traumatic Stress, 11*(1), 3–24. https://doi.org/10.1023/A:1024448814268

Carroll, R. T. (n.d.). Eye movement desensitization and reprocessing (EMDR). *The skeptic's dictionary.* http://skepdic.com/emdr.html

Castelli Gattinara, P., Onofri, A., & Angelini, C. (2017). The EMDR approach used as a tool to provide psychological help to refugees and asylum seekers. In M. Nickerson (Ed.), *Cultural competence and healing culturally based trauma with EMDR therapy: Innovative strategies and protocols* (pp. 129–144). Springer.

Chang, S. C. (2017). EMDR therapy as affirmative care for transgender and gender nonconforming clients. In M. Nickerson (Ed.), *Cultural competence and healing culturally based trauma with EMDR therapy: Innovative strategies and protocols* (pp. 177–194). Springer.

Chemtob, C. M., Nakashima, J., & Carlson, J. G. (2002). Brief treatment for elementary school children with disaster-related posttraumatic stress disorder: A field study. *Journal of Clinical Psychology, 58*(1), 99–112. https://doi.org/10.1002/jclp.1131

Chen, Y.-R., Hung, K.-W., Tsai, J.-C., Chu, H., Chung, M.-H., Chen, S.-R., Liao, Y.-M., Ou, K.-L., Chang, Y.-C., & Chou, K.-R. (2014). Efficacy of eye-movement desensitization and reprocessing for patients with posttraumatic-stress disorder: A meta-analysis of randomized controlled trials. *PLOS ONE, 9*(8), Article e103676. https://doi.org/10.1371/journal.pone.0103676

Christman, S. D., Garvey, K. J., Propper, R. E., & Phaneuf, K. A. (2003). Bilateral eye movements enhance the retrieval of episodic memories. *Neuropsychology, 17*(2), 221–229. https://doi.org/10.1037/0894-4105.17.2.221

Cooper, N. A., & Clum, G. A. (1989). Imaginal flooding as a supplementing for PTSD in combat veterans: A controlled study. *Behavior Therapy, 20*(3), 381–391. https://doi.org/10.1016/S0005-7894(89)80057-7

de Bont, P. A. J. M., van den Berg, D. P. G., van der Vleugel, B. M., de Roos, C., de Jongh, A., van der Gaag, M., & van Minnen, A. M. (2016). Prolonged exposure and EMDR for PTSD v. a PTSD waiting-list condition: Effects on symptoms of psychosis, depression and social functioning in patients with chronic psychotic disorders. *Psychological Medicine, 46*(11), 2411–2421. https://doi.org/10.1017/S0033291716001094

Department of Veterans Affairs & Department of Defense. (2004). *VA/DoD clinical practice guideline for the management of post-traumatic stress* (Office of Quality and Performance publication 10Q-CPG/PTSD-04). Veterans Health Administration, Department of Veterans Affairs and Health Affairs, Department of Defense.

Department of Veterans Affairs & Department of Defense. (2017). *VA/DoD clinical practice guidelines for the management of post-traumatic stress* (Office of Quality and Performance publication 10Q-CPG/PTSD-17). Veterans Health Administration, Department of Veterans Affairs and Health Affairs, Department of Defense.

de Roos, C., Greenwald, R., den Hollander-Gijsman, M., Noorthoorn, E., van Buuren, S., & de Jongh, A. (2011). A randomised comparison of cognitive behavioural therapy (CBT) and eye movement desensitisation and reprocessing (EMDR) in disaster-exposed children. *European Journal of Psychotraumatology, 2*(1), 5694–5704. https://doi.org/10.3402/ejpt.v2i0.5694

de Roos, C., van der Oord, S., Zijlstra, B., Lucassen, S., Perrin, S., Emmelkamp, P., & de Jongh, A. (2017). Comparison of eye movement desensitization and reprocessing therapy, cognitive behavioral writing therapy, and wait-list in pediatric posttraumatic stress disorder following single-incident trauma: A multicenter randomized clinical trial. *Journal of Child Psychology and Psychiatry, and Allied Disciplines, 58*(11), 1219–1228. https://doi.org/10.1111/jcpp.12768

Devilly, G. J., & Spence, S. H. (1999). The relative efficacy and treatment distress of EMDR and a cognitive-behavior trauma treatment protocol in the amelioration of posttraumatic stress disorder. *Journal of Anxiety Disorders, 13*(1–2), 131–157. https://doi.org/10.1016/S0887-6185(98)00044-9

Diehle, J., Opmeer, B. C., Boer, F., Mannarino, A. P., & Lindauer, R. J. (2015). Trauma-focused cognitive behavioral therapy or eye movement desensitization and reprocessing: What works in children with posttraumatic stress symptoms? A randomized controlled trial. *European Child & Adolescent Psychiatry, 24*(2), 227–236. https://doi.org/10.1007/s00787-014-0572-5

Dominguez, S. K., & Lee, C. W. (2017, August 22). Errors in the 2017 APA clinical practice guideline for the treatment of PTSD: What the data actually says. *Frontiers in Psychology.* https://doi.org/10.3389/fpsyg.2017.01425

Edmond, T., & Rubin, A. (2004). Assessing the long-term effects of EMDR: Results from an 18-month follow-up study with adult female survivors of CSA. *Journal of Child Sexual Abuse, 13*(1), 69–86. https://doi.org/10.1300/J070v13n01_04

Ehring, T., Welboren, R., Morina, N., Wicherts, J. M., Freitag, J., & Emmelkamp, P. M. G. (2014). Meta-analysis of psychological treatments for posttraumatic stress disorder in adult survivors of childhood abuse. *Clinical Psychology Review, 34*(8), 645–657. https://doi.org/10.1016/j.cpr.2014.10.004

El Khoury-Malhame, M., Lanteaume, L., Beetz, E. M., Roques, J., Reynaud, E., Samuelian, J.-C., Blin, O., Garcia, R., & Khalfa, S. (2011). Attentional bias in post-traumatic stress disorder diminishes after symptom amelioration. *Behaviour Research and Therapy, 49*(11), 796–801. https://doi.org/10.1016/j.brat.2011.08.006

Elofsson, U. O. E., von Schèele, B., Theorell, T., & Söndergaard, H. P. (2008). Physiological correlates of eye movement desensitization and reprocessing. *Journal of Anxiety Disorders, 22*(4), 622–634. https://doi.org/10.1016/j.janxdis.2007.05.012

EMDRIA. (n.d.). *EMDR certification.* https://www.emdria.org/emdr-training-education/emdr-certification/

Fernandez, I. (2007). EMDR as a treatment of post-traumatic reactions: A field study on child victims of an earthquake [Special issue]. *Educational and Child Psychology Therapy, 24,* 65–72.

Forbes, D., Bisson, J. I., Monson, C. M., & Berliner, L. (2020). *Effective treatments for PTSD: Practice guidelines from the International Society for Traumatic Stress Studies* (3rd ed.). Guilford Press.

Galatzer-Levy, I. R., Nickerson, A., Litz, B. T., & Marmar, C. R. (2013). Patterns of lifetime PTSD comorbidity: A latent class analysis. *Depression and Anxiety, 30*(5), 489–496. https://doi.org/10.1002/da.22048

Gil-Jardiné, C., Evrard, G., Al Joboory, S., Tortes Saint Jammes, J., Masson, F., Ribéreau-Gayon, R., Galinski, M., Salmi, L.-R., Revel, P., Régis, C. A., Valdenaire, G., & Lagarde, E. (2018). Emergency room intervention to prevent post concussion-like symptoms and post-traumatic stress disorder: A pilot randomized controlled study of a brief eye movement desensitization and reprocessing intervention versus reassurance or usual care. *Journal of Psychiatric Research, 103,* 229–236. https://doi.org/10.1016/j.jpsychires.2018.05.024

Gomez, A. (2013). *EMDR therapy and adjunct approaches with children: Complex trauma, attachment, and dissociation.* Springer.

Haerizadeh, M., Sumner, J. A., Birk, J. L., Gonzalez, C., Heyman-Kantor, R., Falzon, L., Gershengoren, L., Shapiro, P., & Kronish, I. M. (2020). Interventions for posttraumatic stress disorder symptoms induced by medical events: A systematic review. *Journal of Psychosomatic Research, 129*, Article 109908. https://doi.org/10.1016/j.jpsychores.2019.109908

Harris, H., Urdaneta, V., Triana, V., Vo, C. S., Walden, D., & Myers, D. (2018). A pilot study with Spanish-speaking Latina survivors of domestic violence comparing EMDR & TFCBT group interventions. *Open Journal of Social Sciences, 6*(11), 203–222. https://doi.org/10.4236/jss.2018.611015

Hartung, J. (2017). Teaching and learning EMDR in diverse countries and cultures. When to start, what to do, when to leave. In M. Nickerson (Ed.), *Cultural competence and healing culturally based trauma with EMDR therapy: Innovative strategies and protocols* (pp. 323–340). Springer.

Hase, M., Plagge, J., Hase, A., Braas, R., Ostacoli, L., Hofmann, A., & Huchzermeier, C. (2018). Eye movement desensitization and reprocessing versus treatment as usual in the treatment of depression: A randomized-controlled trial. *Frontiers in Psychology, 9*, 1384. https://doi.org/10.3389/fpsyg.2018.01384.

Herbert, J. D., Lilienfeld, S. O., Lohr, J. M., Montgomery, R. W., O'Donohue, W. T., Rosen, G. M., & Tolin, D. F. (2000). Science and pseudoscience in the development of eye movement desensitization and reprocessing: Implications for clinical psychology. *Clinical Psychology Review, 20*(8), 945–971. https://doi.org/10.1016/S0272-7358(99)00017-3

Hertlein, K. M., & Ricci, R. J. (2004). A systematic research synthesis of EMDR studies: Implementation of the platinum standard. *Trauma, Violence & Abuse, 5*(3), 285–300. https://doi.org/10.1177/1524838004264340

Ho, M. S. K., & Lee, C. W. (2012). Cognitive behaviour therapy versus eye movement desensitization and reprocessing for post-traumatic disorder— Is it all in the homework then? *European Review of Applied Psychology/Revue Européenne de Psychologie Appliquée, 62*(4), 253–260. https://doi.org/10.1016/j.erap.2012.08.001.

Högberg, G., Pagani, M., Sundin, O., Soares, J., Aberg-Wistedt, A., Tärnell, B., & Hällström, T. (2008). Treatment of post-traumatic stress disorder with eye movement desensitization and reprocessing: Outcome is stable in 35-month follow-up. *Psychiatry Research, 159*(1–2), 101–108. https://doi.org/10.1016/j.psychres.2007.10.019

Houben, S. T. L., Otgaar, H., Roelofs, J., Merckelbach, H., & Muris, P. (2020). The effects of eye movements and alternative dual tasks on the vividness and emotionality of negative autobiographical memories: A meta-analysis of laboratory studies. *Journal of Experimental Psychopathology*. Advance online publication. https://doi.org/10.1177/2043808720907744

Hudson, J. I., Chase, E. A., & Pope, H. G., Jr. (1998). Eye movement desensitization and reprocessing in eating disorders: Caution against premature acceptance. *The International Journal of Eating Disorders, 23*(1), 1–5. https://doi.org/10.1002/(SICI)1098-108X(199801)23:1<1::AID-EAT1>3.0.CO;2-Q

Hurley, E. C. (2018). Effective treatment of veterans with PTSD: Comparison between intensive daily and weekly EMDR approaches. *Frontiers in Psychology, 9*, 1458. https://doi.org/10.3389/fpsyg.2018.01458

Hyer, L., & Brandsma, J. M. (1997). EMDR minus eye movements equals good psychotherapy. *Journal of Traumatic Stress, 10*(3), 515–522. https://doi.org/10.1002/jts.2490100314

Ichii, M., & Ohtsuka, M. (2014, January 9–10). *EMDR history in Japan. In EMDR: Social and cultural adaptations/integration with other therapies* [Paper presentation]. EMDR Asia International Conference, Manila, The Philippines. https://emdria.omeka.net/items/show/22576

Institute of Medicine. (2007). *Treatment of posttraumatic stress disorder: An assessment of the evidence*. National Academies Press.

Ironson, G., Freund, B., Strauss, J. L., & Williams, J. (2002). Comparison of two treatments for traumatic stress: A community-based study of EMDR and prolonged exposure. *Journal of Clinical Psychology, 58*(1), 113–128. https://doi.org/10.1002/jclp.1132

Ironson, G., Hylton, E., Gonzalez, B., Small, B., Freund, B., Gerstein, M., Thurston, F., & Bira, L. (2021). Effectiveness of three brief treatments for recent traumatic events in a low-SES community setting. *Psychological Trauma: Theory, Research, Practice, and Policy*. Advance online publication. https://doi.org/10.1037/tra0000594

Isomaa, R., Backholm, K., & Birgegård, A. (2015). Posttraumatic stress disorder in eating disorder patients: The roles of psychological distress and timing of trauma. *Psychiatry Research, 230*(2), 506–510. https://doi.org/10.1016/j.psychres.2015.09.044

Jaberghaderi, N., Greenwald, R., Rubin, A., Dolatabadim, S., & Zand, S. O. (2004). A comparison of CBT and EMDR for sexually abused Iranian girls. *Clinical Psychology & Psychotherapy, 11*(5), 358–368. https://doi.org/10.1002/cpp.395

Jarero, I., Givaudan, M., & Osorio, A. (2018). Randomized controlled trial on the provision of the EMDR integrative group treatment protocol adapted for ongoing traumatic stress to female patients with cancer-related posttraumatic stress disorder symptoms. *Journal of EMDR Practice and Research, 12*(3), 94–104. https://doi.org/10.1891/1933-3196.12.3.94

Jarero, I. N., Uribe, S., Artigas, L., & Givaudan, M. (2015). EMDR protocol for recent critical incidents: A randomized controlled trial in a technological disaster context. *Journal of EMDR Practice and Research, 9*(4), 166–173. https://doi.org/10.1891/1933-3196.9.4.166

Jayatunge, R. M. (2006). *The efficacy of EMDR: A study based on Sri Lankan combatants.* EMDR Humanitarian Assistance Program.

Jayatunge, R. M. (2013, December). Treating mild traumatic brain injury with EMDR. *Lanka Web.* http://www.lankaweb.com/news/items/2013/12/18/treating-mild-traumatic-brain-injury-with-emdr/

Jeffries, F. W., & Davis, P. (2013). What is the role of eye movements in eye movement desensitization and reprocessing (EMDR) for post-traumatic stress disorder (PTSD)? A review. *Behavioural and Cognitive Psychotherapy, 41*(3), 290–300. https://doi.org/10.1017/S1352465812000793

Jensen, J. A. (1994). An investigation of eye movement desensitization and reprocessing (EMD/R) as a treatment for posttraumatic stress disorder (PTSD) symptoms of Vietnam combat veterans. *Behavior Therapy, 25*(2), 311–325. https://doi.org/10.1016/S0005-7894(05)80290-4

John-Baptiste Bastien, R., Jongsma, H. E., Kabadayi, M., & Billings, J. (2020). The effectiveness of psychological interventions for post-traumatic stress disorder in children, adolescents and young adults: A systematic review and meta-analysis. *Psychological Medicine, 50*(10), 1598–1612. https://doi.org/10.1017/S0033291720002007

Kane, J. C., Adaku, A., Nakku, J., Odokonyero, R., Okello, J., Musisi, S., Augustinavicius, J., Greene, M. C., Alderman, S., & Tol, W. A. (2015). Challenges for the implementation of World Health Organization guidelines for acute stress, PTSD, and bereavement: A qualitative study in Uganda. *Implementation Science, 11*, Article 36. https://doi.org/10.1186/s13012-016-0400-z

Karatzias, T., Murphy, P., Cloitre, M., Bisson, J., Roberts, N., Shevlin, M., Hyland, P., Maercker, A., Ben-Ezra, M., Coventry, P., Mason-Roberts, S., Bradley, A., & Hutton, P. (2019). Psychological interventions for ICD-11 complex PTSD symptoms: Systematic review and meta-analysis. *Psychological Medicine, 49*(11), 1761–1775. https://doi.org/10.1017/S0033291719000436

Kazdin, A. E. (2005). Treatment outcomes, common factors, and continued neglect of mechanisms of change. *Clinical Psychology: Science and Practice, 12*(2), 184–188. https://doi.org/10.1093/clipsy.bpi023

Keane, T. M. (1998). Psychological and behavioral treatment of posttraumatic stress disorder. In P. Nathan & J. Gorman (Eds.), *Guide to treatments that work* (pp. 398–407). Oxford University Press.

Kemp, M., Drummond, P., & McDermott, B. (2010). A wait-list controlled pilot study of eye movement desensitization and reprocessing (EMDR) for children with post-traumatic stress disorder (PTSD) symptoms from motor vehicle accidents. *Clinical Child Psychology and Psychiatry, 15*(1), 5–25. https://doi.org/10.1177/1359104509339086

Knipe, J. (2015). *EMDR toolbox: Theory and treatment of complex PTSD and dissociation.* Springer.

Korn, D. L., & Leeds, A. M. (2002). Preliminary evidence of efficacy for EMDR resource development and installation in the stabilization phase of treatment of complex posttraumatic stress disorder. *Journal of Clinical Psychology, 58*(12), 1465–1487. https://doi.org/10.1002/jclp.10099

Korn, D. L., Maxfield, L., Smyth, N. J., & Stickgold, R. (2017). *EMDR Fidelity Rating Scale (EFRS).* https://emdrfoundation.org/research-grants/emdr-fidelity-rating-scale/

Kuiken, D., Bears, M., Miall, D., & Smith, L. (2001). Eye movement desensitization reprocessing facilitates attentional orienting. *Imagination, Cognition and Personality, 21*(1), 3–20. https://doi.org/10.2190/L8JX-PGLC-B72R-KD7X

Landin-Romero, R., Novo, P., Vicens, V., McKenna, P. J., Santed, A., Pomarol-Clotet, E., Salgado-Pineda, P., Shapiro, F., & Amann, B. L. (2013). EMDR therapy modulates the default mode network in a subsyndromal, traumatized bipolar patient. *Neuropsychobiology, 67*(3), 181–184. https://doi.org/10.1159/000346654

Lansing, K., Amen, D. G., Hanks, C., & Rudy, L. (2005). High-resolution brain SPECT imaging and eye movement desensitization and reprocessing in police officers with PTSD. *The Journal of Neuropsychiatry and Clinical Neurosciences, 17*(4), 526–532. https://doi.org/10.1176/jnp.17.4.526

Laugharne, J., Kullack, C., Lee, C. W., McGuire, T., Brockman, S., Drummond, P. D., & Starkstein, S. (2016). Amygdala volumetric change following psychotherapy for posttraumatic stress disorder. *The Journal of Neuropsychiatry and Clinical Neurosciences, 28*(4), 312–318. https://doi.org/10.1176/appi.neuropsych.16010006

Lee, C., Gavriel, H., Drummond, P., Richards, J., & Greenwald, R. (2002). Treatment of PTSD: Stress inoculation training with prolonged exposure compared to EMDR. *Journal of Clinical Psychology, 58*(9), 1071–1089. https://doi.org/10.1002/jclp.10039

Lee, C. W., & Cuijpers, P. (2013). A meta-analysis of the contribution of eye movements in processing emotional memories. *Journal of Behavior Therapy and Experimental Psychiatry, 44*(2), 231–239. https://doi.org/10.1016/j.jbtep.2012.11.001

Lee, C. W., & Cuijpers, P. (2014). What does the data say about the importance of eye movement in EMDR? *Journal of Behavior Therapy and Experimental Psychiatry, 45*(1), 226–228. https://doi.org/10.1016/j.jbtep.2013.10.002

Lee, C. W., de Jongh, A., & Hase, M. (2019). Lateral eye movements, EMDR, and memory changes: A critical commentary on Houben et al. (2018). *Clinical Psychological Science, 7*(3), 403–404. https://doi.org/10.1177/2167702619830395

Lee, C. W., & Schubert, S. (2009). Omissions and errors in the Institute of Medicine's report on scientific evidence of treatment for posttraumatic stress disorder. *Journal of EMDR Practice and Research, 3*(1), 32–38. https://doi.org/10.1891/1933-3196.3.1.32

Lee, C. W., Taylor, G., & Drummond, P. D. (2006). The active ingredient in EMDR: Is it traditional exposure or dual focus of attention? *Clinical Psychology & Psychotherapy, 13*(2), 97–107. https://doi.org/10.1002/cpp.479

Leeds, A. M. (2009). *A guide to the standard EMDR protocols for therapists, supervisors, and consultants.* Springer.

Leeds, A. M. (2016). *A guide to the standard EMDR therapy protocols for therapists, supervisors, and consultants* (2nd ed.). Springer.

Leer, A., Engelhard, I. M., Dibbets, P., & van den Hout, M. A. (2013). Dual-tasking attenuates the return of fear after extinction. *Journal of Experimental Psychopathology, 4*(4), 325–340. https://doi.org/10.5127/jep.029412

Lenferink, L. I. M., Meyerbröker, K., & Boelen, P. A. (2020). PTSD treatment in times of COVID-19: A systematic review of the effects of online EMDR. *Psychiatry Research.* Advance online publication. https://doi.org/10.1016/j.psychres.2020.113438

Lenz, A. S., Haktanir, A., & Callender, K. (2017). Meta-analysis of trauma-focused therapies for treating the symptoms of posttraumatic stress disorder. *Journal of Counseling and Development, 95*(3), 339–353. https://doi.org/10.1002/jcad.12148

Lipke, H. J., & Botkin, A. (1992). Case studies of eye movement desensitization and reprocessing (EMDR) with chronic post-traumatic stress disorder. *Psychotherapy: Theory, Research, & Practice, 29*(4), 591–595. https://doi.org/10.1037/0033-3204.29.4.591

Lipscomb, A., & Ashley, W. (2021). A critical analysis of the utilization of eye movement desensitization and reprocessing (EMDR) psychotherapy with African-American clients. *Journal of Human Services: Training, Research, and Practice, 7*(1), Article 3.

Lohr, J. M., Lilienfeld, S. O., Tolin, D. F., & Herbert, J. D. (1999). Eye movement desensitization and reprocessing: An analysis of specific versus nonspecific treatment factors. *Journal of Anxiety Disorders, 13*(1–2), 185–207. https://doi.org/10.1016/S0887-6185(98)00047-4

Luber, M. (2019). *Treating eating disorders, chronic pain, and maladaptive self-case behaviors: Eye movement desensitization and reprocessing (EMDR) therapy scripted protocols and summary sheets.* Springer.

Lutz, B. (2017). Culturally attuned EMDR therapy with an immigrant woman suffering from social anxiety. In M. Nickerson (Ed.), *Cultural competence and healing culturally based trauma with EMDR therapy: Innovative strategies and protocols* (pp. 113–128). Springer.

Manzoni, M., Fernandez, I., Bertella, S., Tizzoni, F., Gazzola, E., Molteni, M., & Nobile, M. (2021). Eye movement desensitization and reprocessing: The state of the art of efficacy in children and adolescent with post traumatic stress disorder. *Journal of Affective Disorders, 282,* 340–347. https://doi.org/10.1016/j.jad.2020.12.088

Marcus, S., Marquis, P., & Sakai, C. (2004). Three-and 6-month follow-up of EMDR treatment of PTSD in an HMO setting. *International Journal of Stress Management, 11*(3), 195–208. https://doi.org/10.1037/1072-5245.11.3.195

Marcus, S. V., Marquis, P., & Sakai, C. (1997). Controlled study of treatment of PTSD using EMDR in an HMO setting. *Psychotherapy: Theory, Research, & Practice, 34*(3), 307–315. https://doi.org/10.1037/h0087791

Masters, R., McConnell, E., & Juhasz, J. (2017). Learning EMDR in Uganda: An experiment in cross cultural collaboration. In M. Nickerson (Ed.), *Cultural competence and healing culturally based trauma with EMDR therapy: Innovative strategies and protocols* (pp. 305–323). Springer.

Maxfield, L., & Hyer, L. (2002). The relationship between efficacy and methodology in studies investigating EMDR treatment of PTSD. *Journal of Clinical Psychology, 58*(1), 23–41. https://doi.org/10.1002/jclp.1127

Mbazzi, F. B., Dewailly, A., Admasu, K., Duagani, Y., Wamala, K., Vera, A., Bwesigye, D., & Roth, G. (2021). Cultural adaptations of the standard EMDR protocol in five African countries. *Journal of EMDR Practice and Research, 15*(1), 29–43. https://doi.org/10.1891/EMDR-D-20-00028

McLay, R. N., Webb-Murphy, J. A., Fesperman, S. F., Delaney, E. M., Gerard, S. K., Roesch, S. C., Nebeker, B. J., Pandzic, I., Vishnyak, E. A., & Johnston, S. L. (2016). Outcomes from eye movement desensitization and reprocessing in active-duty service members with posttraumatic stress disorder. *Psychological Trauma: Theory, Research, Practice, and Policy, 8*(6), 702–708. https://doi.org/10.1037/tra0000120

McNally, R. J. (1999). EMDR and Mesmerism: A comparative historical analysis. *Journal of Anxiety Disorders, 13*(1–2), 225–236. https://doi.org/10.1016/S0887-6185(98)00049-8

Merriam-Webster. (n.d.). Proprietary. In *Merriam-Webster.com dictionary.* Retrieved March 11, 2021, from https://www.merriam-webster.com/dictionary/proprietary

Meysner, L., Cotter, P., & Lee, C. W. (2016). Evaluating the efficacy of EMDR with grieving individuals: A randomized control trial. *Journal of EMDR Practice and Research, 10*(1), 2–12. https://doi.org/10.1891/1933-3196.10.1.2

Narimani, M., Ahari, S., & Rajabi, S. (2008). Comparison of efficacy of eye movement, desensitization and reprocessing and cognitive behavioral therapy therapeutic methods for reducing anxiety and depression of Iranian combatant afflicted by post traumatic stress disorder. *Journal of Applied Sciences, 8*(10), 1932–1937. https://doi.org/10.3923/jas.2008.1932.1937

Nickerson, M. (Ed.). (2017a). *Cultural competence and healing culturally based trauma with EMDR therapy: Innovative strategies and protocols.* Springer.

Nickerson, M. (2017b). Dismantling prejudice and exploring social privilege with EMDR therapy. In M. Nickerson (Ed.), *Cultural competence and healing culturally based trauma with EMDR therapy: Innovative strategies and protocols* (pp. 53–76). Springer.

Nickerson, M. (2017c). Healing culturally based trauma and exploring social identities with EMDR therapy. In M. Nickerson (Ed.), *Cultural competence and healing culturally based trauma with EMDR therapy: Innovative strategies and protocols* (pp. 29–52). Springer.

Nickerson, M. (2017d). Integrating cultural concepts and terminology into the AIP model and EMDR approach. In M. Nickerson (Ed.), *Cultural competence and healing culturally based trauma with EMDR therapy: Innovative strategies and protocols* (pp. 15–28). Springer.

Nijdam, M. J., Gersons, B. P. R., Reitsma, J. B., de Jongh, A., & Olff, M. (2012). Brief eclectic psychotherapy v. eye movement desensitisation and reprocessing therapy for post-traumatic stress disorder: Randomised controlled trial. *The British Journal of Psychiatry, 200*(3), 224–231. https://doi.org/10.1192/bjp.bp.111.099234

Niroomandi, R. (2012). Efficacy of eye movement desensitization and reprocessing (EMDR) in the Iranian veterans with chronic posttraumatic stress disorder (PTSD) after Iran/Iraq War. *International Proceedings of Economics Development and Research, 40*, 52–56.

Novo Navarro, P., Landin-Romero, R., Guardiola-Wanden-Berghe, R., Moreno-Alcázar, A., Valiente-Gómez, A., Lupo, W., García, F., Fernández, I., Pérez, V., & Amann, B. L. (2018). 25 years of Eye Movement Desensitization and Reprocessing (EMDR): The EMDR therapy protocol, hypotheses of its mechanism of action and a systematic review of its efficacy in the treatment of post-traumatic stress disorder. *Revista de Psiquiatria y Salud Mental, 11*(2), 101–114. https://doi.org/10.1016/J.RPSMEN.2015.12.002.

O'Brien, J. M. (2017). EMDR therapy with lesbian/gay/bisexual clients. In M. Nickerson (Ed.), *Cultural competence and healing culturally based trauma with EMDR therapy: Innovative strategies and protocols* (pp. 195–208). Springer.

Oh, D.-H., & Choi, J. (2004). Changes in the regional cerebral perfusion after eye movement desensitization and reprocessing: A SPECT study of two cases. *Korean Journal of Biological Psychiatry, 11*(2), 173–180.

Osorio, A., Pérez, M., Tirado, G., Jarero, I., & Givaudan, M. (2018). Randomized controlled trial on the EMDR integrative group treatment protocol for ongoing traumatic stress with adolescents and young adults patients with cancer. *American Journal of Applied Psychology, 7*(4), 50–56. https://doi.org/10.11648/j.ajap.20180704.11

Ost, J. (2006). EMDR: Of limited use, whichever way you look at it. *Healthwatch Newsletter, 58*, 4–5.

Pagani, M., Di Lorenzo, G., Verardo, A. R., Nicolais, G., Monaco, L., Lauretti, G., Russo, R., Niolu, C., Ammaniti, M., Fernandez, I., & Siracusano, A. (2012). Neurobiological correlates of EMDR monitoring—An EEG study. *PLOS ONE, 7*(9), Article e45753. https://doi.org/10.1371/journal.pone.0045753

Pagani, M., Högberg, G., Salmaso, D., Nardo, D., Sundin, O., Jonsson, C., Soares, J., Aberg-Wistedt, A., Jacobsson, H., Larsson, S. A., & Hällström, T. (2007). Effects of EMDR psychotherapy on 99mTc-HMPAO distribution in occupation-related post-traumatic stress disorder. *Nuclear Medicine Communications, 28*(10), 757–765. https://doi.org/10.1097/MNM.0b013e3282742035

Parker, A., Buckley, S., & Dagnall, N. (2009). Reduced misinformation effects following saccadic bilateral eye movements. *Brain and Cognition, 69*(1), 89–97. https://doi.org/10.1016/j.bandc.2008.05.009

Parnell, L. (2006). *A therapist's guide to EMDR: Tools and techniques for successful treatment.* Norton.

Peters, E., Wissing, M. P., & Du Plessis, W. F. (2002). Implementation of EMDR(R) with cancer patients: Research. *Health South Africa Gesondheld, 7*(2), 100–109. https://hdl.handle.net/10520/EJC35219

Pineles, S. L., Shipherd, J. C., Mostoufi, S. M., Abramovitz, S. M., & Yovel, I. (2009). Attentional biases in PTSD: More evidence for interference. *Behaviour Research and Therapy, 47*(12), 1050–1057. https://doi.org/10.1016/j.brat.2009.08.001

Pitman, R. K., Orr, S. P., Altman, B., Longpre, R. E., Poiré, R. E., & Macklin, M. L. (1996). Emotional processing during eye movement desensitization and reprocessing therapy of Vietnam veterans with chronic posttraumatic stress disorder. *Comprehensive Psychiatry, 37*(6), 419–429. https://doi.org/10.1016/S0010-440X(96)90025-5

Power, K. G., McGoldrick, T., Brown, K., Buchanan, R., Sharp, D., Swanson, V., & Karatzias, A. (2002). A controlled comparison of eye movement desensitization and reprocessing versus exposure plus cognitive restructuring versus waiting list in the treatment of post-traumatic stress disorder. *Journal of Clinical Psychology and Psychotherapy, 9*(5), 299–318. https://doi.org/10.1002/cpp.341

Rahimi, F., Rejeh, N., Bahrami, T., Heravi-Karimooi, M., Tadrisi, S. D., Griffiths, P., & Vaismoradi, M. (2019). The effect of the eye movement desensitization and reprocessing intervention on anxiety and depression among patients undergoing hemodialysis: A randomized controlled trial. *Perspectives in Psychiatric Care, 55*(4), 652–660. https://doi.org/10.1111/PPC.12389

Rogers, S., Silver, S., Goss, J., Obenchain, J., Willis, A., & Whitney, R. (1999). A single session, group study of exposure and eye movement desensitization and reprocessing in treating posttraumatic stress disorder among Vietnam War veterans: Preliminary data. *Journal of Anxiety Disorders, 13*, 119–130. https://doi.org/10.1016/S0887-6185(98)00043-7

Rostaminejad, A., Behnammoghadam, M., Rostaminejad, M., Behnammoghadam, Z., & Bashti, S. (2017). Efficacy of eye movement desensitization and reprocessing on the phantom limb pain of patients with amputations within a 24-month follow-up. *International Journal of Rehabilitation Research/Internationale Zeitschrift fur Rehabilitationsforschung/Revue Internationale de Recherches de Readaptation, 40*(3), 209–214. https://doi.org/10.1097/MRR.0000000000000227

Rothbaum, B. O. (1997). A controlled study of eye movement desensitization and reprocessing in the treatment of posttraumatic stress disordered sexual assault victims. *Bulletin of the Menninger Clinic, 61*(3), 317–334.

Rothbaum, B. O., Astin, M. C., & Marsteller, F. (2005). Prolonged exposure versus eye movement desensitization and reprocessing (EMDR) for PTSD rape victims. *Journal of Traumatic Stress, 18*(6), 607–616. https://doi.org/10.1002/jts.20069

Rousseau, P.-F., Boukezzi, S., Garcia, R., Chaminade, T., & Khalfa, S. (2020). Cracking the EMDR code: Recruitment of sensory, memory and emotional networks during bilateral alternating auditory stimulation. *The Australian and New Zealand Journal of Psychiatry, 54*(8), 818–831. https://doi.org/10.1177/0004867420913623

Rousseau, P.-F., El Khoury-Malhame, M., Reynaud, E., Boukezzi, S., Cancel, A., Zendjidjian, X., Guyon, V., Samuelian, J.-C., Guedj, E., Chaminade, T., & Khalfa, S. (2019). Fear extinction learning improvement in PTSD after EMDR therapy: An fMRI study. *European Journal of Psychotraumatology, 10*(1), Article 1568132. https://doi.org/10.1080/20008198.2019.1568132

Russell, M. C. (2006). Treating combat-related stress disorders: A multiple case study utilizing eye movement desensitization and reprocessing (EMDR) with battlefield casualties from the Iraqi war. *Military Psychology, 18*(1), 1–18. https://doi.org/10.1207/s15327876mp1801_1

Russell, M. C. (2008a). Scientific resistance to research, training and utilization of eye movement desensitization and reprocessing (EMDR) therapy in treating post-war disorders. *Social Science & Medicine, 67*(11), 1737–1746. https://doi.org/10.1016/j.socscimed.2008.09.025

Russell, M. C. (2008b). Treating traumatic amputation-related phantom limb pain: A case study utilizing eye movement desensitization and reprocessing (EMDR) within the armed services. *Clinical Case Studies, 7*(2), 136–153. https://doi.org/10.1177/1534650107306292

Russell, M. C. (2008c). War-related medically unexplained symptoms, prevalence and treatment: Utilizing EMDR within the armed services. *Journal of EMDR Practice and Research, 2*(2), 212–225. https://doi.org/10.1891/1933-3196.2.3.212

Russell, M. C., & Figley, C. R. (2013). *Treating traumatic stress disorders in military personnel: An EMDR practitioner's guide.* Routledge. https://doi.org/10.4324/9780203829721

Russell, M. C., & Friedberg, F. (2009). Training, treatment access and research on trauma intervention in the armed services. *Journal of EMDR Practice and Research, 3*(1), 24–31. https://doi.org/10.1891/1933-3196.3.1.24

Russell, M. C., Lipke, H. E., & Figley, C. R. (2019). EMDR therapy. In B. A. Moore & W. A. Penk (Eds.), *Handbook for the treatment of PTSD in military personnel* (pp. 78–94). Guilford Press.

Russell, M. C., Silver, S. M., Rogers, S., & Darnell, J. N. (2007). Responding to an identified need: A joint DoD-DVA training program in EMDR for therapists providing trauma services. *International Journal of Stress Management, 14*(1), 61–71. https://doi.org/10.1037/1072-5245.14.1.61

Scheck, M. M., Schaeffer, J. A., & Gillette, C. (1998). Brief psychological intervention with traumatized young women: The efficacy of eye movement desensitization and reprocessing. *Journal of Traumatic Stress, 11*(1), 25–44. https://doi.org/10.1023/A:1024400931106

Schneider, J., Hofmann, A., Rost, C., & Shapiro, F. (2008). EMDR in the treatment of chronic phantom limb pain. *Pain Medicine, 9*(1), 76–82. https://doi.org/10.1111/j.1526-4637.2007.00299.x

Schubert, S. J., Lee, C. W., & Drummond, P. D. (2011). The efficacy and psychophysiological correlates of dual-attention tasks in eye movement desensitization and reprocessing (EMDR). *Journal of Anxiety Disorders, 25*(1), 1–11. https://doi.org/10.1016/j.janxdis.2010.06.024

Seidler, G. H., & Wagner, F. E. (2006). Comparing the efficacy of EMDR and trauma-focused cognitive-behavioral therapy in the treatment of PTSD:

A meta-analytic study. *Psychological Medicine, 36*(11), 1515–1522. https://doi.org/10.1017/S0033291706007963

Shapiro, E., & Laub, B. (2015). Early EMDR intervention following a community critical incident: A randomized clinical trial. *Journal of EMDR Practice and Research, 9*(1), 17–27. https://doi.org/10.1891/1933-3196.9.1.17

Shapiro, F. (1989). Efficacy of the eye movement desensitization procedure in the treatment of traumatic memories. *Journal of Traumatic Stress, 2*(2), 199–223. https://doi.org/10.1002/jts.2490020207

Shapiro, F. (1995). *Eye movement desensitization and reprocessing: Basic principles, protocols, and procedures.* Guilford Press.

Shapiro, F. (2018). *Eye movement desensitization and reprocessing (EMDR) therapy: Basic principles, protocols, and procedures* (3rd ed.). Guilford Press.

Shapiro, F., Russell, M. C., Lee, C., & Schubert, S. (2020). Eye movement desensitization and reprocessing therapy. In D. Forbes, J. Bisson, C. Monson and L. Berliner (Eds.), *Effective treatments for PTSD: Practice guidelines from the International Society for Traumatic Stress Studies* (3rd ed., pp. 234–254). Guilford Press.

Shapiro, R. (2017). EMDR with issues of appearance, aging, and class. In M. Nickerson (Ed.), *Cultural competence and healing culturally based trauma with EMDR therapy: Innovative strategies and protocols* (pp. 295–302). Springer.

Sheikhi, M., Moradi, M., Shahsavary, S., Alimoradi, Z., & Salimi, H. R. (2020). The effect of eye movement desensitization and reprocessing on the fear of hypoglycemia in type 2 diabetic patients: A randomized clinical trial. *BMC Psychology, 8*(1), Article 82. https://doi.org/10.1186/s40359-020-00450-0

Silver, S. M., Brooks, A., & Obenchain, J. (1995). Treatment of Vietnam War veterans with PTSD: A comparison of eye movement desensitization and reprocessing, biofeedback, and relaxation training. *Journal of Traumatic Stress, 8*(2), 337–342. https://doi.org/10.1002/jts.2490080212

Silver, S. M., & Rogers, S. (2002). *Light in the heart of darkness: EMDR and the treatment of war and terrorism survivors.* Norton.

Silver, S. M., Rogers, S., Knipe, J., & Colelli, G. (2005). EMDR therapy following the 9/11 terrorist attacks: A community-based intervention project in New York City. *International Journal of Stress Management, 12*(1), 29–42. https://doi.org/10.1037/1072-5245.12.1.29

Silver, S. M., Rogers, S., & Russell, M. (2008). Eye movement desensitization and reprocessing (EMDR) in the treatment of war veterans. *Journal of Clinical Psychology, 64*(8), 947–957. https://doi.org/10.1002/jclp.20510

Smyth-Dent, K., Fitzgerald, J., & Hagos, Y. (2019). A field study of the EMDR integrative group treatment protocol for ongoing traumatic stress provided to adolescent Eritrean refugees living in Ethiopia. *Psychology and Behavioral Science International Journal, 12*(4), 1–12.

Stickgold, R. (2002). EMDR: A putative neurobiological mechanism of action. *Journal of Clinical Psychology, 58*(1), 61–75. https://doi.org/10.1002/jclp.1129

Substance Abuse and Mental Health Services Administration. (2010, October). *Eye movement desensitization and reprocessing.* National Registry of Evidence-Based Programs and Practices, U.S. Department of Health and Human Services.

Susanty, E., Sijbrandij, M., Srisayekti, W., & Huizink, A. C. (2021). Eye movement desensitization (EMD) to reduce posttraumatic stress disorder-related stress reactivity in Indonesia PTSD patients: A study protocol for a randomized controlled trial. *Trials, 22*(1), 181. https://doi.org/10.1186/s13063-021-05100-3

Suzuki, A., Josselyn, S. A., Frankland, P. W., Masushige, S., Silva, A. J., & Kida, S. (2004). Memory reconsolidation and extinction have distinct temporal and biochemical signatures. *The Journal of Neuroscience, 24*(20), 4787–4795. https://doi.org/10.1523/JNEUROSCI.5491-03.2004

Taylor, S., Thordarson, D. S., Maxfield, L., Fedoroff, I. C., Lovell, K., & Ogrodniczuk, J. (2003). Comparative efficacy, speed, and adverse effects of three PTSD treatments: Exposure therapy, EMDR, and relaxation training. *Journal of Consulting and Clinical Psychology, 71*(2), 330–338. https://doi.org/10.1037/0022-006x71.2.330

ter Heide, F. J. J., Mooren, T. M., Kleijn, W., de Jongh, A., & Kleber, R. J. (2011). EMDR versus stabilisation in traumatised asylum seekers and refugees: Results of a pilot study. *European Journal of Psychotraumatology, 2*(1), Article 5881. https://doi.org/10.3402/ejpt.v2i0.5881

ter Heide, F. J. J., Mooren, T. M., van de Schoot, R., de Jongh, A., & Kleber, R. J. (2016). Eye movement desensitisation and reprocessing therapy v. stabilisation as usual for refugees: Randomised controlled trial. *The British Journal of Psychiatry, 209*(4), 311–318. https://doi.org/10.1192/bjp.bp.115.167775

Tesarz, J., Leisner, S., Gerhardt, A., Janke, S., Seidler, G. H., Eich, W., & Hartmann, M. (2014). Effects of eye movement desensitization and reprocessing (EMDR) treatment in chronic pain patients: A systematic review. *Pain Medicine, 15*(2), 247–263. https://doi.org/10.1111/pme.12303

Thomaes, K., Engelhard, I. M., Sijbrandij, M., Cath, D. C., & Van den Heuvel, O. A. (2016). Degrading traumatic memories with eye movements: A pilot functional MRI study in PTSD. *European Journal of Psychotraumatology, 7*(1), Article 31371. https://doi.org/10.3402/ejpt.v7.31371

Thompson, C. T., Vidgen, A., & Roberts, N. P. (2018). Psychological interventions for post-traumatic stress disorder in refugees and asylum seekers: A systematic review and meta-analysis. *Clinical Psychology Review, 63*, 66–79. https://doi.org/10.1016/j.cpr.2018.06.006

U.S. Department of Veterans Affairs. (2020). *Eye movement desensitization and reprocessing (EMDR) for PTSD.* https://www.ptsd.va.gov/understand_tx/emdr.asp

van den Berg, D., de Bont, P. A. J. M., van der Vleugel, B. M., de Roos, C., de Jongh, A., van Minnen, A., & van der Gaag, M. (2018). Long-term outcomes of trauma-focused treatment in psychosis. *The British Journal of Psychiatry, 212*(3), 180–182. https://doi.org/10.1192/bjp.2017.30

van den Berg, D. P. G., de Bont, P. A. J. M., van der Vleugel, B. M., de Roos, C., de Jongh, A., Van Minnen, A., & van der Gaag, M. (2015). Prolonged exposure vs eye movement desensitization and reprocessing vs waiting list for post-traumatic stress disorder in patients with a psychotic disorder: A randomized clinical trial. *JAMA Psychiatry, 72*(3), 259–267. https://doi.org/10.1001/jamapsychiatry.2014.2637

van der Kolk, B. A., Spinazzola, J., Blaustein, M. E., Hopper, J. W., Hopper, E. K., Korn, D. L., & Simpson, W. B. (2007). A randomized clinical trial of eye movement desensitization and reprocessing (EMDR), fluoxetine, and pill placebo in the treatment of posttraumatic stress disorder: Treatment effects and long-term maintenance. *The Journal of Clinical Psychiatry, 68*(1), 37–46. https://doi.org/10.4088/JCP.v68n0105

van Rood, Y. R., & de Roos, C. (2009). EMDR in the treatment of medically unexplained symptoms: A systematic review. *Journal of EMDR Practice and Research, 3*(4), 248–263. https://doi.org/10.1891/1933-3196.3.4.248

van Veen, S. C., van Schie, K., van de Schoot, R., van den Hout, M. A., & Engelhard, I. M. (2020). Making eye movements during imaginal exposure leads to short-lived memory effects compared to imaginal exposure alone. *Journal of Behavior Therapy and Experimental Psychiatry.* Advance online publication. https://doi.org/10.1016/j.jbtep.2019.03.001

Vaughan, K., Armstrong, M. S., Gold, R., O'Connor, N., Jenneke, W., & Tarrier, N. (1994). A trial of eye movement desensitization compared to image habituation training and applied muscle relaxation in post-traumatic stress disorder. *Journal of Behavior Therapy and Experimental Psychiatry, 25*(4), 283–291. https://doi.org/10.1016/0005-7916(94)90036-1

Venkatraman, L. R., & Siniego, L. (2017). An integrative approach to EMDR therapy as an anti-oppression endeavor. In M. Nickerson (Ed.), *Cultural competence and healing culturally based trauma with EMDR therapy: Innovative strategies and protocols* (pp. 79–96). Springer.

Wesson, M., & Gould, M. (2009). Intervening early with EMDR on military operations. *Journal of EMDR Practice and Research, 3*(2), 91–97. https://doi.org/10.1891/1933-3196.3.2.91

Wilson, S. A., Becker, L. A., & Tinker, R. H. (1995). Eye movement desensitization and reprocessing (EMDR) treatment for psychologically traumatized individuals. *Journal of Consulting and Clinical Psychology, 63*(6), 928–937. https://doi.org/10.1037/0022-006X.63.6.928

Wilson, S. A., Becker, L. A., & Tinker, R. H. (1997). Fifteen-month follow-up of eye movement desensitization and reprocessing (EMDR) treatment for posttraumatic stress disorder and psychological trauma. *Journal of Consulting and Clinical Psychology, 65*(6), 1047–1056. https://doi.org/10.1037/0022-006X.65.6.1047

Wolpe, J., & Abrams, J. (1991). Post-traumatic stress disorder overcome by eye-movement desensitization: A case report. *Journal of Behavior Therapy and Experimental Psychiatry, 22*(1), 39–43. https://doi.org/10.1016/0005-7916(91)90032-Z

World Health Organization. (2013). *Guidelines for the management of conditions specifically related to stress.* https://apps.who.int/iris/bitstream/handle/10665/85119/9789241505406_eng.pdf;jsessionid=F5EB3E2FB9A36EA3B0B150BCA86C454F?sequence=1

World Health Organization. (2019). *International statistical classification of diseases and related health problems.* https://www.who.int/standards/classifications/classification-of-diseases

Wright, S. A., & Russell, M. C. (2013). Treating violent impulses: A case study utilizing eye movement desensitization and reprocessing with a military client. *Clinical Case Studies, 12*(2), 128–144. https://doi.org/10.1177/1534650112469461

Yunitri, N., Kao, C. C., Chu, H., Voss, J., Chiu, H. L., Liu, D., Shen, S. H., Chang, P.-C., Kang, X. L., & Chou, K.-R. (2020). The effectiveness of eye movement desensitization and reprocessing toward anxiety disorder: A meta-analysis of randomized controlled trials. *Journal of Psychiatric Research, 123*, 102–113. https://doi.org/10.1016/j.jpsychires.2020.01.005

Yurtsever, A., Konuk, E., Akyüz, T., Zat, Z., Tükel, F., Çetinkaya, M., Savran, C., & Shapiro, E. (2018). An eye movement desensitization and reprocessing (EMDR) group intervention for Syrian refugees with post-traumatic stress symptoms: Results of a randomized controlled trial. *Frontiers in Psychology, 9*, 493. https://doi.org/10.3389/fpsyg.2018.00493

Zimmermann, E. (2014). EMDR humanitarian work: Providing trainings in EMDR therapy to African clinicians. *Journal of EMDR Practice and Research, 8*(4), 240–247. https://doi.org/10.1891/1933-3196.8.4.240

Zimmermann, P., Biesold, K. H., Barre, K., & Lanczik, M. (2007). Long-term course of post-traumatic stress disorder (PTSD) in German soldiers: Effects of inpatient eye movement desensitization and reprocessing therapy and specific trauma characteristics in patients with non-combat-related PTSD. *Military Medicine, 172*(5), 456–460. https://doi.org/10.7205/MILMED.172.5.456

Index

Abrams, J., 13
Abreaction, 169
Abuse, sexual, 122, 125
Accelerated reprocessing, 73–78
Active listening, 136
Adaptive information processing (AIP)
    about, 25, 36
    and cultural diversity, 38–39
    defined, 169
    on early trauma and adverse childhood experiences, 48
    EMDR based on, 25–26
    explaining, for client preparation, 54–55
    mechanisms of action, 32–35
    principles, 26–29
    psychopathology and resilience, 30–31
    traumatic stressors blocking, 28–29
Adaptive neural networks, 31
Adolescents, 108–111, 123
Affect scan, 50–51, 169
Affect tolerance, 44, 57
Africa, 117–120
African American clients, 116
Agitation, severe, 45

AIP. *See* Adaptive information processing
Alliance, therapeutic. *See* Therapeutic alliance
Alternating tapping, 56–57
Alternating vibration pads, 57
American Psychiatric Association, 105–106
American Psychological Association (APA), 9, 18
Amygdala, 34
Antioch University Seattle, 131
Anxiety, 87, 90
APA (American Psychological Association), 9, 18
Artigas, L., 117
Ashley, W., 115
Assessment (phase 3), 61–86
    about, 5, 61
    case example, 62, 161–163
    image selection, 62–64
    negative cognition identification, 64–66
    Standard Protocol Worksheet, 140–141
Associative processing, 76–77
Attachment, 29
Attention, dual-focused, 32–33, 170

Auditory sounds
  bilateral stimulation using, 56
  cerebral hemispheres activated
      with, 33
  sensory memories experienced
      through, 63

Behaviors
  high-risk, 53
  maladaptive, 30
  pathologic, 30
Beliefs, blocking. See Blocking beliefs
Between-session changes, 95–96
Between-session logs, 94–95
Biases, negative attentional, 32
Bilateral stimulation (BLS)
  changing mechanics of, 82–83
  with children and adolescents,
      109–110
  defined, 29, 169
  EMDR as alternative to, 43
  eye movement for, 72–73
  intrinsic information processing
      system activated by, 29
  introducing, to clients, 55–56
  as mechanism of action, 33–35, 115
  techniques for, 56–57
  use of, in Africa, 119–120
Biofeedback and relaxation training, 103
Bipolar disorder, 45
Blocked reprocessing, 78, 80–86
Blocking beliefs, 78, 88, 169
BLS. See Bilateral stimulation
Body scan (phase 6), 88–90
  about, 5
  case example, 166
  Standard Protocol Worksheet, 142
Body sensations, identifying, 71–72
Bradley, R., 112–113, 130
Brain
  and lateralization, 33–34
  and mechanisms of action, 34
  plasticity of, 97

Brake and gas pedal metaphor, 59
Brickell, M., 113
Butterfly hug, 57, 110

Cancer, 108, 117
Carlson, J. G., 105
Carroll, R. T., 15
Case example
  assessment (phase 3), 62
  EMDR therapy, 155–168
  of maladaptive neural networks, 31
CBT (cognitive-behavioral therapy),
      106, 122
CBWT (cognitive behavior writing
      therapy), 110
Cerebral hemispheres, 33
Change, stability of, 125
Children, 108–111, 123
Choices, and reprocessing issues, 86
Clients
  explaining role of, 57–58
  history of. See Client history
      [phase 1]
  preparing. See Client preparation
      [phase 2]
Client history (phase 1), 42–53
  about, 5, 42
  case example, 156–159
  client safety and suitability, 42–43
  comorbidities of traumatic stress
      injury, 52–53
  contraindications, 43–46
  current contributors, 47–51
  future contributors, 51–52
  past contributors, 47–51
  three-pronged protocol, 46–47
  treatment planning, 46
Client preparation (phase 2), 53–61
  about, 5
  affect tolerance and safe/calm
      spaces, 57
  body sensation identification,
      71–72

case example, 159–161
client and therapist role
        clarification, 57–58
for CPTSD, 106
EMDR mechanics demonstrations,
        55–57
emotion identification, 69–70
establishing therapeutic alliance,
        54
estimating SUD, 70–71
explaining AIP model, 54–55
introducing metaphor for expected
        client role, 58–59
length and pace of treatment
        sessions, 60–61, 125
positive cognition selection, 66–68
rating validity of cognition, 68–69
resource development and
        installation, 59–60
Standard Protocol Worksheet,
        139–140
Clinical practice guidelines, 6–8
Closure (phase 7), 91–95
    about, 6
    case example, 166
    Standard Protocol Worksheet, 143
Cochrane Review, 103
Cognition
    negative. *See* Negative cognition
    positive. *See* Positive cognition
Cognitive-behavioral therapy (CBT),
        106, 122
Cognitive behavior model, 37
Cognitive behavior writing therapy
        (CBWT), 110
Cognitive interweaves, 83–86, 170
Cognitive model, 37
Cognitive processing therapy (CPT),
        103
Combat stress, 104–105
Comorbidities, 52–53
Complex PTSD (CPTSD), 106
Complex trauma, 105–107

Contraindications, 43–46
Contributors
    current, 51, 157
    future, 51–52
    past. *See* Past contributors
Controversy, 15–17, 22–23, 135
Co-occurring conditions, 111–112
CPT (cognitive processing therapy),
        103
CPTSD (complex PTSD), 106
Culturally diverse populations
    and AIP theory, 38–39
    evaluation with, 115–116
    future directions in studies of, 131
    importance of considering, 115
Current contributors, 51, 157

Davis, P., 33
Debriefing, 94
Democratic Republic of Congo, 117
Depakote (valproate), 45
Department of Defense (DoD), 14, 17,
        52, 102
Department of Veterans Affairs (DVA),
        14, 17, 22, 52, 102
Depression, 111
De Roos, C., 110
Desensitization (phase 4), 72–86
    about, 5, 72–73
    accelerated reprocessing of
        memories, 73–78
    blocked reprocessing, 78
    blocked reprocessing strategies,
        80–86
    case example, 163–165
    intense emotional reprocessing
        management, 78–79
    Standard Protocol Worksheet,
        141–142
Detachment, retinal, 43
*Diagnostic and Statistical Manual of
        Mental Disorders* (DSM-5), 13,
        106, 130

Diehle, J., 110
Discomfort, eye, 43
Disorders
  bipolar, 45
  dissociative, 45
  eating, 129
  seizure, 44
  substance use, 45
Dissemination, proprietary, 19–22, 132
Dissociative disorder, 45
DoD. *See* Department of Defense
DSM-5. *See Diagnostic and Statistical Manual of Mental Disorders*
Dual-focused attention, 32–33, 170
DVA. *See* Department of Veterans Affairs

Earliest–worst–recent reprocessing sequence, 48–49
Early intervention, 107–108
Eating disorders, 129
Ecological validity, 78, 97
Effectiveness, studies of, 112–114
Efficacy, 22, 101–104
Ehring, T., 106
Electronic devices, BLS using, 57
EMD (eye movement desensitization), 4, 12–13
EMDR. *See* Eye movement desensitization and reprocessing
EMDR Humanitarian Assistance Program (HAP), 21, 117, 127
EMDRIA. *See* EMDR International Association
EMDR-IGTP (EMDR integrative group treatment protocol), 117–118
EMDR Institute, 8, 15, 20
EMDR integrative group treatment protocol (EMDR-IGTP), 117–118

EMDR International Association (EMDRIA), 8, 20, 127, 132
EMDR-PRECI, 107–108
EMDR textbook, 20
EMDR Therapy Standard Protocol Worksheet, 139–143
Emotions, 69–70, 162–163
Ethical Principles of Psychologists and Code of Conduct (APA), 9
Ethiopia, 118
Evaluation, 101–125
  in children and adolescents, 108–111
  co-occurring and other psychological conditions, 111–112
  with culturally diverse populations, 115–116
  of delivery and stability of change, 125
  of early intervention, 107–108
  effectiveness research, 112–114
  efficacy research, 101–104
  in international communities, 116–125
  on mechanism of actions, 114–115
  with selected populations, 104–107
Evidence-based treatment, EMDR as, 4–8
Exposure
  as mechanism of action, 35
  prolonged, 103
Eye discomfort, 43
Eye movement desensitization (EMD), 4, 12–13
Eye movement desensitization and reprocessing (EMDR)
  and cultural diversity, 9–10
  eight phases of trauma-focused protocol, 4
  as evidence-based treatment, 4–8
  introduction of, 3–4
  training. *See* Training

Eye Movement Desensitization and Reprocessing (Shapiro), 11, 20

Fatigue, 44
Feeder memories
  about, 50
  defined, 170
  therapist screening for, 50–51
Fernandez, I., 123
First responders, 43–44
Float back techniques, 50, 170
Follow-up sessions, 99–100
Future contributors, 51–52
Future research directions, 127–133

Gestalt model, 37
Gil-Jardiné, C., 108
Great Hanshin Earthquake, 120
Grief, 51
Gustatory, 64

HAP. *See* EMDR Humanitarian Assistance Program
Hartung, J., 9–10
Health concerns, 44
High-risk behaviors, 53
Hippocampus, 34
History, 11–23
  controversy and resistance, 15–17
  mechanism of action, 18–19
  origins, 12–14
  paradigm shift, 14–15
  and perpetuating controversy today, 22–23
  proprietary dissemination, 19–22
  PTSD management guidelines, 17–18
Hostility, 45
Houben, S. T. I., 32
Hug, butterfly, 57, 110
Humanistic model, 37
Hurley, E., 114

Ichii, Masaya, 120–121
Image selection
  in assessment (phase 3), 62–64
  case example, 162
Imminent pending dangerous missions, 43–44
Incomplete sessions, 92–94
Indonesia, 121
Information processing system
  intrinsic, 29
Installation (phase 5), 86–88
  about, 5
  case example, 165–166
  Standard Protocol Worksheet, 142
Institute of Medicine (IOM), 22
Intense emotional reprocessing, 78–79
International communities, 116–125
International guidelines, 8
International Society for Traumatic Stress Studies (ISTSS), 102
International Statistical Classification of Diseases and Related Health Problems, 106
Intervention, early, 107–108
Intoxication, 81
Intrinsic information processing system, 26–29
IOM (Institute of Medicine), 22
Iran, 122–123
Ironson, G., 115
"I" statements
  and negative cognition, 65
  for positive cognition, 66
ISTSS (International Society for Traumatic Stress Studies), 102
Italy, 123

Japan, 120–121
Japanese Journal of EMDR Research and Practice, 120–121
Jarero, I., 123
Jayatunge, R. M., 124
Jeffries, F. W., 33
Journal of Traumatic Stress, 14

Kaiser Permanente, 125
Kane, J. C., 117
Kazdin, Alan, 19
Keane, Terence, 16
Kemp, M., 111
Kenya, 118
Kinesthetic stimuli, 33, 56–57
Korn, D. I., 106–107
Korn, Debra, 59

Lateralization, 33
Law enforcement, 43–44
Lee, C. W., 32
Leeds, Andrew, 29, 44, 59, 106–107, 120
Legal considerations, 46
Liberty City, Florida, 115
Light bars, 56
Lipke, Howard, 17
Lipscomb, A., 115
Listening, active, 136
Lithium, 45
Logs, between-session, 94–95

Maladaptive behaviors, 30
Maladaptive neural networks, 31
Marcus, S., 60
Marquis, Priscilla, 56
Masters, R., 117
Mastery resources, 60
Mbazzi, F. B., 117–118
McNally, Richard, 15
Mechanisms of action, 32–35
    bilateral stimulation, 33–34
    dual-focused attention, 32–33
    evaluation on, 114–115
    exposure as, 35
    historical theories of, 18–19
Medical concerns, 44
Medications, 45
Memories
    clusters of, 48
    feeder. *See* Feeder memories

and intrinsic information
        processing system, 28
    networks of, 25–26
    sensory, 62–63
    target. *See* Target memory
Metaphors, for expected client role,
    58–59
Mexico, 123–124
Mild TBI (mTBI), 44, 53
Military personnel, 43–44, 113, 124.
    See also Veterans
Mindful noticing, 58
Molestation, 89–90
mTBI (mild TBI), 44, 53
Muscle tightening, 72

National Center for PTSD (Veterans
    Affairs), 18–19, 128
National Institute for Clinical
    Excellence (UK), 102
National Institute of Mental Health
    (NIMH), 23, 103
NC. *See* Negative cognition
Negative attentional bias, 32
Negative cognition (NC)
    case example, 162
    defined, 170
    identifying, 64–66
    sample of, 153–154
Neural networks
    adaptive, 31
    adaptive associations of, 35–36
    maladaptive, 31
    of memory, 25
    and positive cognition, 66–67
Neurobiological model, 37
Neurodevelopmental conditions,
    128–129
Neuroscience, 130
Nickerson, Mark, 9–10, 38–39
NIMH (National Institute of Mental
    Health), 23, 103
Node, 170

Non-PTSD conditions, 128–129
No response, 80–82
Noticing, mindful, 58

Ohtsuka, M., 120–121
Olfaction, 63–64
Onset, questions to identify, 47–48
Overresponse, 80

Pain, 53
Paraphrasing, 75
Participant cluster, 49
Past contributors
    case example, 158
    complaint and symptom history,
        47–48
    considerations for selecting, 49–50
    earliest–worst–recent reprocessing
        sequence, 48–49
    feeder memories, 50–51
Pathologic behaviors, 30
PC. See Positive cognition
PE (prolonged exposure), 103
Performance anxiety, 90
Peters, E., 117
Phantom limb pain (PLP), 68
Physical symptoms, 89. See also Body
    sensations
Plateaus, 79, 83–84
PLP (phantom limb pain), 68
Positive cognition (PC)
    case example, 162
    defined, 170
    and installation, 87
    sample of, 153–154
    selecting, 66–68
    and VOC, 68
Posttraumatic stress disorder (PTSD)
    in children and adolescents, 109
    clinical practice guidelines, 6–8
    comorbidities with, 52–53
    complex, 106
    EMD for, 4

head-to-head treatment for,
    102–103
Pregnancy, 45
Prolonged exposure (PE), 103
Proprietary dissemination, 19–22, 132
Psychodynamic model, 37
Psychopathology
    and resilience, 30–31
    severe, as contraindication, 45
Psychoses, 45, 112
Psychotherapy research, questions
    of, 101
Psychotropic medications, 45
PTSD. See Posttraumatic stress
    disorder

Rahimi, F., 123
Randomized controlled trials (RCTs),
    128–129
Rapid eye movement (REM) sleep, 55
RDI (resource development and
    installation), 59–60, 149–151
Recent critical incidents, 107–108
Reevaluation (phase 8), 95–100
    about, 6
    case example, 166–167
    Standard Protocol Worksheet, 143
Refugees, 124–125
Relationship resources, 60
Relaxation training, 103
REM (rapid eye movement) sleep, 55
Reprocessing
    accelerated, 73–78
    blocked, 78, 80–86
    fear of, 81
    intense emotional, 78–79
    problems related to, 81–82
    suitability for, 42
    therapist-related factors interfering
        with, 82
Reprocessing sequence, 48–49
Republic of Germany, 124
Resilience, 30–31

Resistance, 15–17
Resolution
  defined, 170
  reevaluating target memory for,
    97–98
Resource development and
    installation (RDI), 59–60,
    149–151
Resources
  mastery, 60
  relationship, 60
  symbolic, 60
Responsibility, 85–86
Retinal detachment, 43
Rostaminejad, A., 122
Rothbaum, Barbara, 103–104
Rousseau, P. -F., 34

Safe and calm spaces
  and affect tolerance, 57
  case example, 160–161
  exercise protocol, 145–147
Safety
  and reprocessing issues, 86
  of space. See Safe and calm spaces
  and suitability, 42–43
Satisfaction surveys, 133
Scans
  affect, 50–51, 169
  body. See Body scan [phase 6]
Seizure disorders, 44
Self-reporting
  of between-session changes, 95–96
  importance of monitoring, 54
  therapist responses to, 75–76
Self-training, 20
Sensory memory, 62–63
Severe agitation, 45
Severe psychopathology, 45
Sexual abuse, 103, 122, 125
Shapiro, Francine, 14, 15, 46, 120
Silver, Steven M., 21, 102–103
Social anxiety, 87

Somatic sensations. See Body
    sensations
South Africa, 117
Sri Lanka, 124
Stability of change, 125
Stimuli
  kinesthetic, 33, 56–57
  visual, 56
Stop signal, 58–59
Stress
  combat and war, 104–105
  and traumatic stress injury, 52–53
Subjective units of disturbance (SUD)
  about, 13
  and ecological validity, 78
  estimating, 70–71
Substance use disorder, 45
SUD. See Subjective units of
    disturbance
Suicidality, 45
Suitability, client safety and, 42–43
Surveys, satisfaction, 133
Susanty, E., 121
Symbolic resources, 60
Syrian refugees, 124–125

Taiwan National Science Council, 111
Talk therapy, 37–38
Taps, 56–57
Target, defined, 170
Target memory
  assessing, 61
  case example, 161–162
  and client history, 42
  reevaluating, 96–98
TBI (traumatic brain injury), 44–45
Telehealth, 131
Terminating therapy, 98–99
TF-CBT (trauma-focused CBT), 103,
    109
Theory, 25–39
  and adaptive associations of neural
    networks, 35–36

AIP. *See* Adaptive information processing
comparative approaches to, 36–37
importance of, 36
of therapeutic relationships, 37–38
Therapeutic alliance
  with African American clients, 116
  establishing, 54
  importance of, 38
  issues in, 43
  skills for forming, 136
Therapists
  functions of, 36
  responses from, 75–76
  role of, clarifying, 57–58
  trust of. *See* Trust
Therapy
  cognitive-behavioral, 106, 122
  cognitive behavior writing, 110
  cognitive processing, 103
  process of. *See* Therapy process
  talk, 37–38
  terminating, 98–99
Therapy process, 41–100, 119
  about, 4, 5–6
  assessment (phase 3), 61–86
  body scan (phase 6), 88–90
  client history (phase 1), 42–53
  client preparation (phase 2), 53–61
  closure (phase 7), 91–95
  desensitization (phase 4), 72–86
  installation (phase 5), 86–88
  reevaluation (phase 8), 95–100
  terminating, 98–99
Three-pronged protocol, 46–47, 170
TICES strategies, 83, 94–95
Timing
  and closure phase, 91
  issues of, 43
Touchstone events, 30

Training, 8–9, 20, 131–133
Transparency, 116
Trauma. *See also* Posttraumatic stress disorder
  complex, 105–107
  explaining, to clients, 54–55
  and resilience, 30
  sexual, 103
Trauma-focused CBT (TF-CBT), 103, 109
Traumatic brain injury (TBI), 44–45
Traumatic stress injury, 52–53
Treatment
  closing sessions of, 91–94
  length and pace of, 60–61
  planning, 46
  process of. *See* Therapy process
Treatment sessions
  closure of. *See* Closure [phase 7]
  evaluating changes between, 95–96
  follow-up, 99–100
  incomplete, 92–94
Triggers
  about, 51
  case example, 158–159
  evaluating new, 98
Trotter, Wilfred, 11
Trust, 38, 43, 136
Turkey, 124–125

Uganda, 118
Underresponse, 80–82
U.S. Navy, 113

VA (Veterans Affairs), 105, 128
Validity, ecological, 78, 97
Validity of cognition (VOC)
  case example, 162
  and installation, 87–88
  rating, 68–69
  use of, 13
Valproate (Depakote), 45
VA Medical Center, Great Lakes, 17

Van der Kolk, B. A., 107
Van Veen, S. C., 34–35
Veterans, 13, 22, 102–103, 105, 113
Veterans Affairs (VA), 105, 128
Vibrations, kinesthetic, 56–57
Visual stimulus, bilateral stimulation
    using, 56
VOC. *See* Validity of cognition

War stress, 104–105
WHO. *See* World Health Organization
Wolpe, Joseph, 12, 13, 16
World Health Organization (WHO),
    8, 17, 106, 108

Zimbabwe, 118
Zimmermann, E., 117

About the Authors

Mark C. Russell, PhD, ABPP, is a core faculty member at Antioch University Seattle and the establishing director of the Institute of War Stress Injury, Recovery, and Social Justice. As a graduate student at Pacific Graduate School of Psychology (now Palo Alto University), he became Francine Shapiro's research assistant and was primarily responsible for developing the theory underlying eye movement desensitization and reprocessing (EMDR). Dr. Russell is a retired navy commander and military psychologist with over 26 years of military service. He became the first certified military EMDR trainer in the Department of Defense and organized a series of just-in-time EMDR trainings for over 265 mental health providers in response to a growing military mental health crisis. He is dual board certified by the American Board of Professional Psychology in clinical psychology and clinical child and adolescent psychology. Dr. Russell has authored over 13 articles and six book chapters on EMDR. He is the coauthor with Dr. Charles R. Figley of *Treating Traumatic Stress Injuries in Military Personnel: An EMDR Practitioner's Guide* (2013) and *Psychiatric Casualties: How and Why the Military Ignores the Full Cost of War* (2021). Dr. Russell is a recognized expert on war stress injuries and was featured in *USA Today* (2007) and the documentary film *Thank You for Your Service* (2015), produced by Tom Donahue. He was awarded the Distinguished Psychologist Award by the Washington State Psychological Association for his sustained effort to transform military mental health care, including advocating for EMDR training and treatment access, as well as the 2018 Award for Outstanding Service to the Field of Trauma Psychology by American Psychological Association Division 56 (Trauma Psychology).

Francine Shapiro, PhD, the originator and developer of eye movement desensitization and reprocessing (EMDR) therapy, was Senior Research Fellow Emeritus at the Mental Research Institute in Palo Alto, California, and executive director of the EMDR Institute in Watsonville, California. She founded and was President Emeritus of the Trauma Recovery/EMDR Humanitarian Assistance Programs, a nonprofit organization that coordinates disaster response and pro bono training worldwide. She was a recipient of the International Sigmund Freud Award for distinguished contribution to psychotherapy, presented by the City of Vienna in conjunction with the World Council for Psychotherapy; the Award for Outstanding Contributions to Practice in Trauma Psychology from Division 56 (Trauma Psychology) of the American Psychological Association; and the Distinguished Scientific Achievement in Psychology Award from the California Psychological Association. Dr. Shapiro was designated as one of the "Cadre of Experts" of the American Psychological Association and the Canadian Psychological Association Joint Initiative on Ethnopolitical Warfare and served as advisor to a wide variety of trauma treatment and outreach organizations and journals. She was an invited speaker at psychology conferences worldwide and wrote and coauthored more than 90 articles, chapters, and books about EMDR. Francine Shapiro died on June 16, 2019. The level of Dr. Shapiro's dedication to advancing EMDR is evidenced by the fact that she continued to work on this book within days before her passing. Survivors of trauma across the world, their families and friends, and their healers alike owe an eternal debt of gratitude to Dr. Shapiro.

About the Series Editor

Matt Englar-Carlson, PhD, is a professor of counseling and director of the Center for Boys and Men at California State University–Fullerton. A Fellow of the American Psychological Association (APA), Dr. Englar-Carlson's scholarship focuses on training helping professionals to work more effectively with boys and men across the full range of human diversity. His publications and presentations are focused on men and masculinities, social justice and diversity issues in psychological training and practice, and theories of psychotherapy. Dr. Englar-Carlson coedited the books *In the Room With Men: A Casebook of Therapeutic Change, Counseling Troubled Boys: A Guidebook for Professionals, Beyond the 50-Minute Hour: Therapists Involved in Meaningful Social Action*, and *A Counselor's Guide to Working With Men*, and he was featured in the APA-produced video *Engaging Men in Psychotherapy*. He was named Researcher of the Year, Professional of the Year, and he received the Professional Service award from the Society for the Psychological Study of Men and Masculinities, and was one of the core authors of the *APA Guidelines for Professional Psychological Practice With Boys and Men*. As a clinician, Dr. Englar-Carlson has worked with children, adults, and families in school, community, and university mental health settings. He is the coauthor of *Adlerian Psychotherapy*, which is part of the Theories of Psychotherapy Series.